SAVING LIVES
The Role Of The Pharmacist In HIV

Saving Lives
The Role Of The Pharmacist In HIV
by Michelle J. Sherman, RPh, FASCP, FACA, AAHIVP

Second Edition

ISBN 978-1490937502

Copyright © 2013-2017
MichRx Pharmacist Consulting Services, Inc.

Limits of Liability and Disclaimer of Warranty
The author and publisher shall not be liable for your misuse of this material. This book is strictly for informational and educational purposes.

MichRx Pharmacist Consulting Services, Inc.
34145 Pacific Coast Hwy #211
Dana Point, CA 92629
888-661-4403; Fax: 509-271-6579
E-mail: SavingLivesBook@MichRxConsulting.com
www.MichRxConsulting.com

Book and book cover design by Jean Boles
jean.bolesbooks@gmail.com

Saving Lives

The Role Of The Pharmacist In HIV

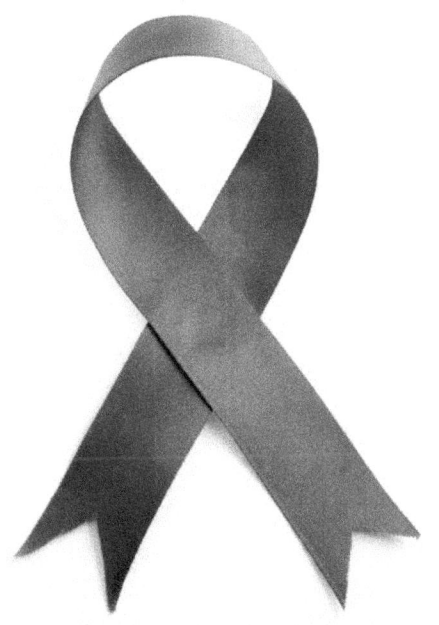

by Michelle J. Sherman,
RPh, FASCP, FACA, AAHIVP

Dedication

This book is dedicated to the hundreds of HIV/AIDS Patients
that I have lost over the past twenty-five years,
and to the hundreds more who fight the fight every single day of your lives.
Your struggle, bravery and courage propel me in the work that I do every day.

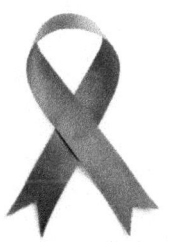

*"In life you can never do a kindness too soon
because you never know how soon it will be too late"*

– Ralph Waldo Emerson

Contents

Endorsements for *Saving Lives* and Michelle Sherman

I opened this book out of curiosity and could not put it down. This book is filled with useful information, made more memorable by powerful examples of good and bad behaviors taken from real-life experiences. This book would be valuable to patients and care-providers alike, but should be required reading for all pharmacy and tech students.

- Dr. Ronald Sherman, MD

~~~~~~

Saving Lives is a must read if you know anyone with HIV. Very well written with very good insights that everyone with HIV should know.

- Rolf Magener

~~~~~~

Michelle Sherman is likely the most well-informed and passionate HIV pharmacist on the planet! She has an uncanny ability to convey complex information in a succinct and understandable manner. This book will prove to be immensely helpful to anyone who wants to be fully informed about effective treatment of HIV. Her book is a "fast-read" and contains several links to credible and invaluable resources for those wanting more specific details.

- Happy-Helper

~~~~~

It has been wonderful to work with Michelle! She is a great resource of information when I put patients on complicated drug regimens or when patients have questions about their medications. She has done research on various herbal and nutritional supplements and their interactions with HIV medications. She has been instrumental in getting patients to understand the importance of adherence, when other providers have failed.

Michelle is enthusiastic, approachable and truly devoted to our patients. She is a respected expert in the field of HIV, and has been teaching in various clinics and pharmacies throughout California about HIV treatment and its complicating illnesses."

- Laura Salazar, MD, AAHIVS

~~~~~

So well written and timely.

 - Don Honan

~~~~~

"I have worked with Michelle Sherman for over 17 years in the field of HIV Medicine. My patients have benefited from her expertise by avoiding side effects, toxicities and adverse drug interactions. I admire her knowledge of complimentary care products. Feedback from patients is very positive, and her experience with anti-viral

Endorsements for *Saving Lives* and Michelle Sherman

medications makes her a valuable resource for patients and physicians alike."

- Korey S. Jorgensen MD
Former Director of HIV Services at The Laguna Beach Community Clinic

~~~~

"Michelle Sherman has been an Assistant Clinical Professor of Pharmacy at UCSF School of Pharmacy for more than 10 years. Her innovative pharmacy practice rotation equips students with the knowledge and skills to help patients with HIV manage their complex medication regimens. More importantly, Michelle is role model clinician and mentor who demonstrates on a daily basis the importance of quality healthcare with a personal touch."

- Robin L. Corelli, Pharm.D.
Professor of Clinical Pharmacy,
Department of Clinical Pharmacy, School of
Pharmacy University of California, San Francisco

~~~~

"Michelle Sherman is known as an HIV pharmacy expert throughout Southern California. I have had the pleasure of working with her for over a decade in multiple settings: specialty pharmacies, academic and public health clinics, and the lecture hall. She has counseled many of my patients regarding their medications, especially regarding adherence and the use of alternative herbal remedies.

13

Through her advocacy and compassion, she has earned the respect of the community. Michelle organizes educational lectures for providers and is a popular speaker herself. Whenever I have a question regarding HIV drug interactions and safety, Michelle is the first person I call. The patients and physicians of Orange County are fortunate to have her as a resource."

- Catherine Diamond MD MPH
Associate Professor of Clinical Medicine
University of California Irvine

~~~~~

"Mich's pharmacology consults are consistently brilliant. Her knowledge in the HIV field is incomparable, where drug interactions and side effects are innumerable. I urge you to use her service, whatever your question or problem....I do!

- Tom Lochner, MD
Newport Beach, CA

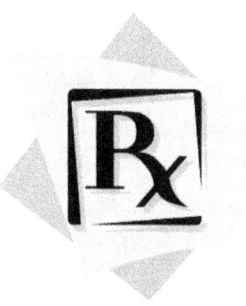

Chapter One:
Saving Lives: My Story

"Those who bring sunshine into the lives of others cannot keep it from themselves"

– J.M. Barrie

As far back as I can remember, growing up in South Africa, one thing was always obvious to me. It was something that emanated from my core, from my soul, if you will. It was the "knowing" that all human beings are created equal, that we are all the same. I had this overwhelming drive to help people.

As you can imagine, while growing up in apartheid South Africa, the gross injustices done to human beings was evident to me at a very early age. Just because of my color, I lived a life of privilege, with a five star education and access to almost everything, while my counterparts, who were black, lived a life of hell and servitude under the apartheid regime. They were faced with inferior education, had to carry "pass books," and were forced to live in segregated, squalid townships and work at menial jobs for very little wage. This injustice and mistreatment of human beings was wrong, and I knew this from my core. As Nelson Mandela said, *To deny people their human rights is to challenge their very humanity."*

During those years when I was growing up in South Africa, all media was censored. I knew nothing of Nelson Mandela until I moved to the United States of America. Everything about him was withheld from us. I always knew that my life's path and journey would involve helping and caring for people; from deep within, I always knew that I was a healer.

The magic began when I was fifteen years old and I began working in my uncle's pharmacy on Saturdays. I loved it, and I learned about all the medications and helped him with dispensing and compounding. I finally knew what I wanted to do—I WAS GOING TO BE A PHARMACIST! Wow, it was so cool, and I knew that as a pharmacist I could help so many people and make a difference in their lives.

I grew up in a society where the majority of the population were mistreated, could not vote, and were not considered citizens. I always had a burning desire to move to the United States, where everyone is free and can be anything they choose to be. It's the land of opportunity; the American dream is real. After graduating from pharmacy school, I worked in my uncle's pharmacy until I had enough money to make my dream come true. By this time, international sanctions were putting a stranglehold on the South African government, and the uprising against the government was intensifying. The government inflicted brutality on those who "disagreed" with their policies or who were outspoken to the injustices they were subjected to; many were arrested and "disappeared"—it was time for me to go.

I left South Africa with three thousand dollars and two suitcases and headed to the United States, to California, to make my dream come true. When I left South Africa there was no news about AIDS in South Africa, or anywhere else in Africa for that matter. The only thing I knew about AIDS is what was going on in the United States; gay men were dying, and Hollywood actor, Rock Hudson had just died. Practicing as a pharmacist in California, I became horrifyingly aware of the magnitude of the AIDS epidemic, and I had some friends who died from AIDS. I knew immediately that taking care of AIDS patients was my calling, my passion, and NOTHING was going to stop me. This was the reason I became a pharmacist; this was my purpose. Caring for my patients was the core of everything for me.

I knew I had to make a difference, and I began volunteering at Laguna Shanti in Laguna Beach California, a tiny city deeply impacted by the AIDS epidemic. I would visit patients in the hospital or at their home, many alone, as they had been disowned by their families, and a week later they were dead. I was witness to sick and dying gentle souls, who were suffering from the stigma of having AIDS and homophobia, and I knew that treating each patient with respect, love, care, empathy and compassion meant everything to them. As Nelson Mandela said, "AIDS is no longer just a disease; it is a human rights issue."

One thing I have realized through all of this is that *Saving Lives* is not always meant in the literal way. You could "Save Lives" when a person is sick, on hospice and dying, by being there, showing that you care and offering love, care, empathy and compassion so that they can die in peace with dignity and grace.

I created the first HIV Specialty Pharmacy in Orange County California while I was still working for a major chain and saw how deeply the services we provided impacted the lives of our patients. As my career evolved, and I moved from "the chain setting" to Independent Pharmacy, the practice grew and grew, and the impact for patients was enormous. We created our consulting company to expand our vision of care for HIV patients. The journey continues, and the power, courage and strength of all my patients propel me forward to do my work every day.

"When you are able to maintain your own highest standards of integrity—regardless of what others may do—you are destined for greatness."

- Napoleon Hill

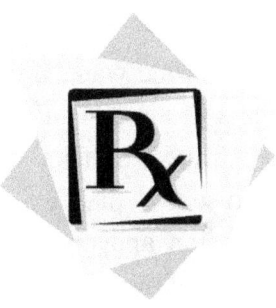

Chapter Two:
Pharmacist as Healthcare Provider

"We make a living by what we get, but we make a life by what we give"

- Winston Churchill

The pharmacist is a healthcare provider. Back in the old days, we had the apothecary—the little old guy standing at the back mixing all his chemicals, potions, tablets and pessaries—or the "druggist" who had the soda fountain in the front end of his store, and he stayed at the back filling the orders from the prescriptions that the physician had written.

We've evolved to the pharmacist of today, who is actually an expert and a specialist in drug utilization and has a vast knowledge about medications, pharmacology and how the medications work. The pharmacist has become the "go to" team member for drug therapy solutions in many settings, and your pharmacy should be NO exception.

If we look at our society, everybody's on a pill for something. Almost everyone wants a quick fix—just take a pill for whatever ails you. You can't sleep, so you take a pill. You can't stay awake, you take another pill. You've got GERD, heart disease, diabetes, high cholesterol, ADD, ADHD, depression and on and on. Many people are on massive amounts of medications.

To compound that, once they've been to their doctor, got their prescription, been to the pharmacy and got their little bag of pills filled, the next thing is they decide they need to take every nutritional supplement, vitamin and everything that's advertised on TV or at the local store as well. There are risks for massive drug interactions and consequences that can be catastrophic, sometimes ultimately resulting in death.

Out of our whole healthcare continuum, with the massive amounts of prescription drugs that our patients use, the pharmacist is absolutely *key*. I refer to myself and my colleagues that I work with as *healthcare providers*. That's what we are. We provide a critical piece. If our area of expertise gets messed up and the patient gets the wrong prescription, if it's not appropriate therapy or they don't understand how to take it, the results can be catastrophic.

Inappropriate medication use costs an estimated $177 billion per year. Everybody's always complaining of the high cost of drugs—especially with the HIV drugs, they cost a fortune. The average cost of an antiretroviral regimen for a healthy HIV patient is around $2500 per month and escalates upwards from there.

Think about what happens with the medications when in the hands of the patient. No matter how expensive those drugs are, what happens on the other end when the patient walks away from your counter with that bag of prescriptions or with prescriptions you've delivered? Do they know what to do or how to take them?

I always use the analogy that the bag of prescriptions that the patient walks away from the counter with is like a loaded gun. It's just like flipping that barrel and playing Russian roulette—when they pull the trigger, they may or may not be shot. Do they know how to take the medication and know if they need to take it with food? Are there drug-drug interactions? Do they understand the adverse reactions they may possibly experience? What other catastrophic results can occur?

This cost of inappropriate medication use amount is massive. Can you imagine if our government had that extra $177 billion? They'd probably be spending it on something else, and we'd still be in the predicament we are, but this is huge. Our cost of healthcare in the United States is just massive. For the most advanced country in the world, our healthcare costs are outrageous.

More than 1.5 million preventable medication-related adverse events occur every year. This number is staggering and is preventable. Has the pharmacist actually spoken with those patients and consulted with them regarding the correct use of the medications and their possible side effects?

When you buy a gun, you've got to know how to use it. These medications are like that as well. A gun could kill you if you don't know what you're doing. So can certain medications. I see it frequently with HIV patients who have been referred to me. The patients may not receive consultations from some of the pharmacies they go to if the pharmacy doesn't specialize in HIV. The pharmacy personnel may not know about the other drugs the patient may be taking. The patient walks away from the counter with a "loaded gun" in their hand, and once they take the medication it's a spin of the barrel; hopefully, the shot doesn't go off.

Here is an example of a recent situation I encountered:

I was doing a talk for HIV clients at a local AIDS Service organization, and when the talk was done, I opened up for questions. One of the clients, a 52-year-old woman who we will call Marjorie, said that she has been on Atripla® for several months and every day she feels exhausted and can barely function and get through the day. My first question to her was, "When do you take the Atripla®?" Her reply was "In the morning, right after I have had breakfast."

Question: "Did your doctor tell you how to take it"?

Answer: "No."

Question: "Do you use an HIV Specialty Pharmacy?"

Answer: "No, because of my insurance, I have to use a chain pharmacy. I use one close to my home."

Question: "Did the pharmacist give you a consultation on the Atripla® when you started it?"

Answer: "No.

There are multitudes of issues going on in this situation that are troublesome, and this was an opportunity for me, as an HIV Specialist Pharmacist and Healthcare Provider, to be able to help Marjorie and improve her situation.

This is how we resolved Marjorie's problem of having possible adverse side effects. This should have been explained by the pharmacist who dispensed the medication to her the first time.

1. I told Marjorie to take the Atripla® at bedtime on an empty stomach instead of in the morning after breakfast. By making this change and taking the Atripla® at bedtime, Marjorie will be sleeping through the majority of the central nervous system side effects, such as dizziness and drowsiness, and she would hopefully be able to function better during the day. If Atripla® is taken with food, absorption increases and the drug levels are increased, resulting in more severe adverse reactions.

2. I informed Marjorie that if there was no improvement and she did not feel better with the

switch, she should go back to her doctor and discuss possible changes in her regimen.

3. Marjorie was also encouraged to seek out an HIV Specialty Pharmacy, if possible, or to make sure she gets consultations on her new medications from the pharmacist.

I saw Marjorie about a month after our discussion, and when I asked her how she was doing, she smiled and said, "I did what you said and started taking the Atripla® at bedtime on an empty stomach and it worked. I feel so much better, it changed my life. Thank you for everything"

My biggest peeve is when clients go to multiple pharmacies. The pharmacists are held hostage because they don't know what the patient is getting elsewhere. There's no continuity in the computer systems. The results could be catastrophic. Always notify your patients that whichever pharmacy they choose, to stay with it and get all of their medications there.

Every dollar spent on pharmacist-patient care services realizes healthcare savings of $16.70. In many states, people have been practicing pharmaceutical or pharmacist care services for many years. This was from a drug-related morbidity and mortality study, updating the cost of illness model, published in the *American Pharmacists Association Journal*. By doing interventions, whether it's in diabetes or asthma, it saved healthcare dollars.

Read "Our Nation's Medication Use Problem" by American Pharmacists Association at this link: http://bit.ly/Spf1Hb, or just scan the QR Code on the following page and get right to the document.

When people complain, "The cost of drugs is so expensive. The pharmacists are making all of the money," obviously they don't know about the ins and outs of pharmacies and how they work. The drugs are very expensive. The reimbursement rates are really low. The overall healthcare costs can be reduced significantly if the patient walks away from the pharmacy counter knowing exactly what to do and how to take their medications.

I make interventions for my patients all the time. When the patient sees the physician, the visit is usually very hurried, as the physician has to see one patient after the next and usually only spends ten to fifteen minutes with each patient. There is a lot to cover in that short amount of time; the patient may just get a prescription from the physician and be sent on their way. The physician may mention side effects with the patient, but it's really up to the pharmacist—the expert in medications—to be able to convey that information to the patient and make sure that they clearly understand what they are taking, why they are taking it, what side effects to be aware of, drug interactions and what to expect. When I sit down and consult with patients, I know that it's so important to go over all the side effects and things that could happen with the medication, so when they walk away, they're armed and know what to expect.

If you don't tell the patient anything and just say, "Just take this with food. Everything will be fine," or even worse, you don't consult with them at all, and then they go home, and it's Saturday morning, the doctor's office is closed, something happens, and they may not be able to reach the pharmacy for some reason. They may get a rash, throw up, get diarrhea or some kind of side effect that makes them really sick. If you haven't prepared them for the possibility of things that could happen, they're just going to stop taking their meds. As we know with antiretrovirals, that can be catastrophic, because they have to take the medicine 95% or greater of the time to prevent drug resistance from developing.

What about hypersensitivity reactions, as in the case with products containing Abacavir. When a patient is unaware of the hypersensitivity reaction and what the symptoms are—perhaps they haven't been consulted by the pharmacist regarding possible symptoms—if they develop symptoms and stop taking the Abacavir instead of calling their doctor, and with the re-challenge with it later, the consequences could be catastrophic and the patient could die.

Drug therapy is at the bull's-eye of treatment strategies for HIV. Pharmacist involvement in the care of HIV infected individuals is critical, especially in the areas of drug therapy counseling, drug interaction monitoring and adherence. In my opinion, we're one of the most important members of an HIV patient's healthcare team. I always use football analogies. I'm going to use one here in the book as well. I always tell the patients they are the quarterback and the rest of their healthcare team—the pharmacist, doctor, case managers, nurses, pharmacy technicians and everybody else who provides care to them—is the rest of their team.

"If you're the patient, you have to throw the football," I tell them. "If you don't tell us, your team members, what is going on with you and be honest with us, we can't have a good plan. We can't catch that pass you throw and we'll never get into the end zone. If your healthcare team does not get into the end zone—that is catastrophic for the quarterback's life. If we're going to the Super Bowl, you don't become MVP. If it's your HIV, it could actually mean a matter of life or death if you don't incorporate your healthcare team."

Pharmacists are critical. Pharmacists are involved in the care of HIV patients. We are the experts in drug therapy management, drug interactions, and side effects. The pharmacist has to be involved, especially in a disease like HIV, where the medications are everything. That's what's keeping our patients alive.

I have been doing this work for over 25 years. The fear and anxiety I see in clients' eyes, every month sometimes—when they have to get their prescriptions—because they are so fearful that, for one reason or another, they might not be able to get their medications. Is their ADAP (AIDS Drug Assistance Program) or health insurance expired? What's going on with their meds? There is such a big focus on it. We, as pharmacists and pharmacy providers, can really alleviate the anxiety and stress that our patients have.

Drug interactions are huge, whether it's vitamins or prescription meds. Monitoring our patients for drug-drug interactions is critical for maintaining good outcomes and quality of life for our patients as well as decreasing healthcare costs. As pharmacists we must be aware of EVERYTHING that our patients are taking, including prescriptions filled at other pharmacies, over the counter medications, vitamins and other supplements and also street drugs. As healthcare providers we have to engage with our patients and ask!

There are many studies that have been published on the value and importance of pharmacists in HIV care in a number of journals.

One study was with Medi-Cal (California Medicaid). It was a pilot program in Los Angeles County where Medi-

Cal reimbursed HIV pharmacies for pharmacist services in providing consultations and making sure the Medi-Cal members knew how to take their medications. For those of you who are unfamiliar with MTM, MTM is medication therapy management. That's what pharmacists as healthcare providers go to school for, to learn how to teach patients how to take their medications, to make those interventions, to call the doctors and make changes to the patients' regimens if necessary.

You can read the entire study at this link: http://bit.ly/WT5ehe, or just scan this QR Code and get right to the document.

As pharmacists we didn't go to school to count in fives and put pills in pill bottles. You can get the entire article if you scan this QR code.

The other study I would like to mention in the book is, ***Kibicho J, Owczarzak J. Pharmacists' strategies for*** *promoting medication adherence among patients with HIV. J Am Pharm Assoc. (2003). 2011 Nov-Dec; 51(6):746-55*

This study showed that pharmacists in community settings went beyond prescription drug counseling mandated by law to provide additional pharmacy services that were tailored to the needs of patients with HIV. Given that many individuals with HIV are living longer, more research is needed on the effectiveness and cost effectiveness of pharmacists' inter-ventions in clinical practice, in order to inform insurance reimbursement policies.

Another study elucidating to the value of HIV Pharmacists is *Pastakia SD, Corbett AH, Raasch RH, Napravnik S, Correll TA. "Frequency of HIV-related medication errors and associated risk factors in hospitalized patients" Ann Pharmacother. 2008 April; 42(4):491-7. Epub 2008 March 18*. This study showed that the alarmingly high frequency of potentially harmful errors uncovered in this study necessitates further investigation using larger sample sizes. Interventions to reduce and prevent these errors must be sought to eliminate the unintended harm associated with hospitalization.

In all three studies mentioned here in the book, pharmacists made a critical impact and difference in the outcomes for HIV patients.

I've worked with the Orange County California area for many years now. I've seen patients in the clinics, provided care and consultations to patients and made a major impact and difference in their outcomes and quality of life.

I presented an Oral Abstract at APhA Annual Meeting and Exposition in Seattle, WA in March 2004. The title of the abstract is "Establishment of Pharmacist Consultation Services and Collaboration between HIV Clinics and a Non Profit Pharmaceutical Care Center Specializing in HIV Care in Orange County, California."

View the entire abstract presentation at this link: http://bit.ly/V2J2LH, or just scan this QR Code and get right to the document.

Another thing I find is when a patient goes to the doctor's office for a visit, they usually only tell the doctor about the drugs that the doctor wrote the prescription for. They're often only in there with the doctor for 10 or 15

minutes. But when they sit down with the pharmacist, it's an entirely different focus. If the patient knows, likes and trusts the pharmacist, they will tell you everything that they're taking. Not only the prescription drugs, but it's also really important to know what supplements and over-the-counter medications they are taking. There are so many drug interactions with the HIV drugs, not only amongst themselves and other prescription drugs but also with supplements, street drugs and other over-the-counter medications.

The pharmacist needs to really build a rapport with the patients so that when you do consult and sit down with them, they will be comfortable and honest enough with you that they will tell you everything. It's that quarterback situation again—the patient being the quarterback. If they tell you every single thing they're taking—street drugs, supplements etc.—you can realize what's going on, why their regimen is failing, or if there are drug interactions. If they omit something and might not tell you they're using meth or cocaine, you and the doctor are scratching your heads. Nobody can figure out what's going on. Again, the patient is not going to get into the end zone. They have to throw the correct pass to their team because we're only as good as the information the patient will give us. If they don't tell us everything, how do you know? You can run every test in the book and scratch your head, but it could be as easy as one question to the client and then they can tell you.

Here is an example:

At one of the clinics I work with, they had a patient who was doing really well. His viral load was undetectable and CD4 count was really good. He was doing well. Then all of a sudden, the CD4 started dropping and the viral load started going up. His physician kept asking him, "Are you taking your medicine?" "Yes. Everything is fine. I take my meds." "Good." Months went by, and the CD4 continued to drop and the viral load continued to rise. He still claimed that he was taking all the medicines. The doctor was doing genotypes, phenotypes and every test available (at a very high cost) to find out what was going on with this person. At one of his visits, he was in the laboratory getting his blood drawn, and he told the medical assistant that he hadn't taken his medicine for three months.

If this patient had been up front and honest with his physician in the first place, it would have averted hundreds of dollars in costs in medical tests. A pharmacist could have effectively nipped this situation in the bud and come up with a solution for him as to why he wasn't taking his medication. Did he just feel sick? Did he just not feel like it? Was he using drugs? Could he not get to the pharmacy to pick up the prescription? What was the reason that he stopped taking his meds? Those are huge interventions that we, as pharmacists, can make.

Another thing that I find interesting is that in many studies on adherence, very often they're looking at pharmacy refills as data. The BIG question I always ask is, *"Just because somebody got a prescription refilled, are they really taking it?"*

Many HIV Specialty pharmacies fill refills automatically for patients each month. What interventions are being made before the refills are filled? Is the pharmacy contacting the patient to see how they are doing and to discuss their refills? In many instances the patient is not contacted on a monthly basis and their refills are just filled, billed and delivered. The patient is getting their refill every 28 or 30 days. It's not really accurate because, are they actually putting the medication in their mouth, and taking it correctly or even taking it at all? Even delivering the prescriptions to their doorstep, are they really taking it? You have to ask them. Are they actually, physically taking those pills out of the bottle, med packs, and bubble packs or however they get it, putting it in their mouth and swallowing it, and are they doing it at the correct time in the correct way?

If patient is doing everything correctly and they are still failing, then there is a whole host of clinical issues that are going on. We have to find out why those drugs aren't getting absorbed or what else is going on.

Studies that look at refill data should be looked at very closely. Which pharmacies did they look at? Did they look at HIV specialty pharmacies, chain stores across the nation or general pharmacies? It's very important to look at where they're getting their data.

Not All Pharmacists Or Pharmacies Are Created Equal

It is so important for our HIV patients to use medical providers who are HIV specialists. An HIV Specialist physician is an expert at treating HIV disease, and the outcomes for the patient are better than if they used a physician who is not an HIV specialist and who has little or no experience treating HIV disease. The same holds true for the patient's pharmacy. The patient's pharmacist and pharmacy need to be an HIV specialist or specialty pharmacy—the outcomes depend on it.

I have been working in HIV for over 20 years. I eat, live and breathe it. Everything about the HIV meds, the disease state and psychosocial issues I have at my fingertips. I'm not a general pharmacist who is dispensing all different types of things every day.

If somebody asked me something about a particular birth control pill or compounded medication they need, I'd have to look it up. I don't do that every day. I work in HIV. The same holds true for any medical provider or pharmacy the patient chooses. It really needs to be an HIV specialist.

Studies have shown that if the medical provider is an HIV specialist, the outcomes of the patients are so much better. That doctor knows what's going on. They have many HIV patients in their practice as opposed to somebody who has a practice on the corner and has one, two or three HIV patients. Over the years, I have seen the reactions patients get from providers that are not HIV specialists or who have very few, if any, HIV patients.

Examples of some of the hurtful comments are the following:

"You just have to take those particular medications because you have HIV. It's your fault that you got it. You just have to deal with it. There's nothing else we can do. Take those medicines. Get sick. Have diarrhea. We can control those."

A patient was referred to a nephrologist. When the doctor walked into the examination room, the patient remarked to the physician that he had AIDS. The doctor abruptly turned around, and as he walked out of the room, he commented, "We do not treat people like you here."

The same holds true with the pharmacies. As an HIV specialist pharmacy, they deal with HIV medicines and drugs all day long as opposed to some small pharmacy somewhere that does not even have the drugs in stock. Many of these pharmacies can't take care of the patients. Often they don't even have the drugs in stock, which is another catastrophic result for the patients. If the drugs aren't in stock, the patient goes without their meds and they are non-adherent. The non-adherence is promoted by the pharmacy, which is a cardinal sin in my book. We're supposed to be promoting adherence, not hindering it for our patients.

The qualifications and credentials of the pharmacists are important. Is the pharmacist and pharmacy staff qualified to be able to provide that consultation and drug therapy management and overall pharmaceutical care needs to the patient?

Are the pharmacies that they go to regular pharmacies or HIV pharmacies? Are the pharmacists in the pharmacy actually HIV specialists? Are the pharmacists actually credentialed in HIV? An HIV expert pharmacist is a pharmacist who has undergone additional or specialized training in HIV, and is an expert in HIV medications, side effects, drug-drug interactions, adherence and other HIV medication related issues. Pharmacists are usually credentialed through the American Academy of HIV Medicine or through an HIV Certification Program at the University Of Buffalo School Of Pharmacy

See American Academy of HIV Medicine at www.aahivm.org, or scan the QR code.

See HIV Certification Program at University of Buffalo School of Pharmacy at http://bit.ly/WTwgoH, or scan the QR code.

What kind of care do the pharmacists provide? Are they just filling, billing and shipping the drugs off to the patient, or are they actually providing care? Are they advocating on behalf of the patient? Are they taking care of the patient who is getting the medication?

All these questions are really important. You've got to be actively involved with the patient. It's not as if the prescription comes along, you just fill it, you look at the label and, thank goodness, there is zero co-pay. That means the insurance worked and you don't have to spend five hours on the phone. Then off it goes to the patient. There is a lot involved.

The pharmacist and pharmacy staff must advocate on behalf of the patient. If a medication is not covered by the patient's insurance company, the pharmacy staff must deal with it. I find that it is important for the patient's stress level to work on the drug prior authorization behind the scenes instead of calling the patient and absolutely freaking them out by saying, "Your drugs aren't covered. Go speak to your doctor, go get another prescription or go figure it out with your insurance." If a pharmacy engages the patient in this way, it completely freaks the patient out. It's too hard for the patient, who is sick, to deal with it, and they usually just say, "I'm not going to get that prescription. I'm done." If the patient does not get the medication that has been prescribed by the physician it can completely compromise their care and outcome.

Here is an example of a pharmacy not advocating for a patient resulting in a negative outcome:

A patient—let's name him Joey—was recently referred to me by a local AIDS Service Organization to assist him with major pharmacy related problems. Joey had been diagnosed with AIDS and had been on an antiretroviral regimen for several months as well as prophylactic treatment for PCP (pneumocystis (carinii) jiroveci, pneumonia and Mac (Mycobacterium Avium Complex), as well as an anti-depressant. He had been under the care of an HIV Specialist physician in a major city, but he had recently relocated and moved to a city in another county.

Joey was on the state Medicaid program, and when he relocated, he moved in with his aunt until such time as he was well enough to move out on his own. He was unfamiliar with the area and access to an HIV specialty pharmacy, so he used the pharmacy nearest his aunt's house, as it was within walking distance. Unfortunately, this pharmacy was a mega giant box store, and the pharmacists and pharmacy staff knew nothing about HIV and antiretroviral medications, and this is where Joey's problems began.

The HIV specialist physician that had been taking care of Joey had provided him with prescriptions so that he could continue his medication without interruption during his relocation and give him time to locate a new physician. The first month the pharmacy eventually filled his prescriptions, but not without incident. When Joey brought the prescriptions to the pharmacy the first time they did not have the medication in stock and he had to go several days without his medication until the drugs arrived at the pharmacy for the pharmacist to dispense. This was the first major problem. Here was a sick patient with AIDS who missed several days of his antiretroviral regimen, and his non-adherence was promoted by the pharmacy because they did not have the medication in stock.

Joey finally picked up his medication from the pharmacy several days later. When the time came for Joey to get refills on his medications again, the problems at the pharmacy got even worse. When Joey moved to the new city in a new county, his Medicaid plan switched to the county's managed care Medicaid program, and in addition, he now had a share of cost spend down on Medicaid. The share of cost spend down for Joey was $800, which means that every month Joey is responsible to pay the first $800 on Medicaid before any medical services such as physicians visits, blood draws, medical tests or prescription drugs would be covered by Medicaid.

When he arrived at the pharmacy, staff told him that his Medicaid did not cover his medications, that he had $800 share of cost and that he had to pay $800 to get his prescriptions. The pharmacy offered no advice for Joey as to what resources are available to assist him; they did not advocate for him or attempt to solve this problem for him in any way. He left the pharmacy without his medications and did not know where to turn. In California, the ADAP program will pay the share of cost amount for qualified individuals. The pharmacy should have known this and been able to provide Joey with information on the ADAP program and how he could become enrolled.

When Joey was referred to me he had been off his medications for three months. To make a bad situation worse, he stopped his antiretroviral medications one by one as he ran out of them, which can lead to antiretroviral resistance. Joey found a new HIV physician but could not see the physician or get his blood work drawn because he had an $800 share of cost. The first time I spoke to Joey, I was able to put his mind at ease and let him know he could get enrolled in the ADAP program to take care of his share of cost. Each month ADAP would pay for $800 worth of his medications and he would then be eligible to have Medicaid pay for all his medical services and remaining prescriptions. He would, of course, have to use an HIV specialty pharmacy that knows what they are doing. With assistance, guidance and advocacy, Joey was able to have his major insurance roadblock explained and handled for him.

He is now back on his medications and able to access his physician and other medical services. Joey now has peace of mind that he will not go without his life-saving medications again, and he has an HIV pharmacist and specialty pharmacy that is taking care of him. *Saving Lives,* that's what being an HIV pharmacist is all about.

As mentioned earlier, providing consultations and educating patients about their medications is very important. They need to know exactly what's in that brown bag when they walk away. Whether they walk away from the pharmacy counter or it gets delivered, they need to know this information. They need to know if there are any changes in their prescriptions. There needs to be follow-ups and continual interaction with the clients on taking the medications. That brown bag is a loaded gun and the patient must know how to use what's in it or the consequences could be fatal.

Each pharmacist encounter with the patient is an opportunity for adherence interventions. Ask the patient, "Are you taking your medicine?" I have had some patients for twenty years and that question, "Are you taking your medicine?" never really gets old. In fact, it's even more important to ask these long-term HIV survivors those questions because they get pill fatigue. Having to take medicine for twenty years every single day with the pressure to never miss a single dose has got to be overwhelming. Many sick people can't even finish a course of antibiotics. Once they start to feel better, they are done with the antibiotics and they stop before the full course is taken.

I see patients that have been really sick with single-digit T-cells coming out of the hospital so critically ill, they are adherent when they go on their meds because they feel so bad. It's when they get better that the work really starts. They say, "I feel better now. Why do I have to take it?" We, as pharmacists, have to teach the patients why that is so important.

We have to advocate for patients if something is not covered by their insurance, as we saw in the earlier example about Joey. The patient may say, "I didn't come and pick up my prescriptions last month because I don't have a car anymore and I didn't have a ride." You can put them in touch with the AIDS service organizations in your community to make sure they get that ride, and the pharmacy could also deliver the medications. They may say that they couldn't get to the doctor's appointment to get a new prescription because they didn't have transportation. The reasons go on and on and we can make a huge difference and help.

The pharmacist is usually much more accessible to patients compared to the physician's office, and oftentimes patients contact us first when a problem arises. Being an expert in HIV and HIV disease allows the pharmacist to solve the problem or direct patients to the physician or community resources to solve the problem. The pharmacist is front and center in the care of HIV patients. If prescriptions aren't covered by insurance, how are we going to get them covered? Can we enroll them in a patient assistance program? Can we get a service organization to pay for it or the co-pays? There is always a way. That's what these specialty pharmacists and pharmacies provide for patients.

**Know Your Pharmacist; Know Your Pharmacy—
Kickbacks And Unethical Behavior**

The role of the pharmacist in HIV is so important. HIV pharmacists are saving lives every day, yet there is the dark side. There are some unscrupulous, uncaring individuals who are opportunists, preying on the sick. Unfortunately, there are these unethical, non-caring people who open so called HIV pharmacies and who prey on the community just to make money. They will say anything and do anything to get patients to use their pharmacies, and to make matters worse, they will obtain medications through unscrupulous means to make even more money.

A kickback is something a pharmacy offers to patients to switch pharmacies and lure them away from their current pharmacy. Kickbacks include things like cell phones, gift cards, iPods, or even paying patients to switch pharmacies. This is an ILLEGAL practice. You name it, it happens—pharmacy owners offering to pay a patient's rent if they come to, or stay at, their pharmacy; undocumented patients being threatened that they will be reported to immigration and Homeland Security. The list goes on and it is a revolting practice. One shady group was so bold as to send skimpy clad guys to sit in another pharmacy's waiting room in order to lure patients to their pharmacy by paying for things for patients and throwing "pool parties." Never once have these patients been told that the pharmacy they are being directed to does not have HIV specialist pharmacists on staff, and in fact, that they know nothing about HIV at all.

Where does the pharmacy purchase medications? Who is their drug wholesaler? Some pharmacies participate in illegal practices and purchase their medications from small wholesalers that obtain medications through illegal means, such as reselling drugs that they get from HIV clients, buying drugs from shady pharmacies or tampering with and repackaging HIV medications. These "shady" wholesalers offer drugs to pharmacies at much lower costs than the pharmacy could buy it for from one of the major drug wholesalers. This drug fraud has resulted in HIV clients getting "used medication" and medications where the meds have been changed and are not the actual medication or dosage that the doctor has prescribed. What the prescription label says and what is actually contained in the bottle are two different things. Getting medications of this kind can be CATASTROPHIC to the patient because:

• The medication has been tampered with and can be contaminated

• It is ILLEGAL to re-use another persons' prescription

• The actual medication in the bottle may be different from what is prescribed, and this can result in failure of the antiretroviral regimen. The contents may be different, or it may be a lower dose or may contain a completely different drug altogether

• The bottle may contain a drug that the patient is allergic to or be a drug that the patient was not prescribed at all, resulting in severe side effects, drug-drug interactions, or even hospitalization and death

Actual examples of this are the following:

- Prezista® 600mg tablet bottle containing Prezista® 300mg tablets inside the bottle

- Combivir® tablets containing Ziagen® tablets inside the bottle

- Zerit® 40mg capsules containing Zerit® 20mg

- Procrit® injections that have been diluted so you don't get the correct dose

Drug fraud and diversion is a major problem, and crackdowns have occurred in New York State as well as other states. There were several pharmacies were the pharmacists were arrested for taking kickbacks. One pharmacist from a major HIV pharmacy took $21 million from using these counterfeit, re-used drugs. These drugs are in the drug supply that our patients are getting. It's a huge problem.

See New York Attorney General Press Release http://bit.ly/To1WwY, or scan the QR code.

I always educate patients. "Know your pharmacist; know your pharmacy." It's a legitimate question for the patients to ask their pharmacy what wholesaler they use. Where do they get their drugs? There are three major wholesalers in the United States that most people use, and those drugs are good drugs. They're coming directly from the manufacturer that all have pedigrees.

The FDA has mandated that drugs have what's called a pedigree so that you can actually trace the drug from the source to the manufacturer and back onto the pharmacy shelves and see where it has been all along the way. Are they using those types of wholesalers or some fly-by-night place that nobody's heard of?

I always tell pharmacists, "If drugs from giant, mega-wholesalers like Cardinal, McKesson or

AmerisourceBergen are more expensive than a tiny wholesaler that you don't even know if the physical building really exists, how can the drugs be cheaper at the tiny place compared to a massive, giant wholesaler?" The pharmacists have to be very careful. That isn't a bad question for clients to ask.

Being proud to be an HIV pharmacist and pharmacy is everything because you are taking care of your patients. You are taking care of a patient with a life-threatening illness where the drug therapy is everything for that patient. It's got to be 100% correct every time. The pharmacist is a healthcare provider, saving lives every day.

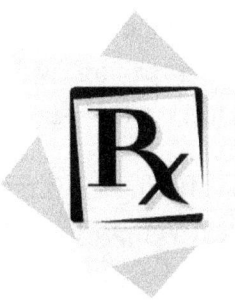

Chapter Three:
HIV Sensitivity

"It is not HIV that is killing us, it is the stigma attached to it."

— Fagmeeda Miller, Positive Muslims, South Africa

The key to having a successful HIV pharmacy and being a successful HIV pharmacist is being HIV sensitive and making sure that all pharmacy staff is trained and is HIV sensitive. Over the years I have heard horror stories, and I still hear them today. For many it is hard to believe that HIV discrimination still exists in this day and age, but I am here to tell you, "Yes, it does."

HIV does not discriminate. The only criteria you need to have this virus is to be a human being. That is all. The Centers for Disease Control has recommended universal HIV testing for people aged 15 to 64. HIV testing is no longer an opt-in test, whereby the patient has to opt in, agree, and sign to get an HIV test. It is now an opt-out test, whereby the patient has to refuse the test and opt out of getting it. HIV testing should now be part of routine medical care. Just as a person would get an annual cholesterol or thyroid test, so they should get an HIV test.

All physicians are not offering universal HIV testing as a matter of routine. When you go to the physician and are not offered an HIV test, they are making a judgment on you. You're not that type of woman or you may not be a gay man. For whatever reason, they don't offer you the test because they think you're not that type of person. If you have human DNA, you should be getting an HIV test. It doesn't matter how old you are, what color you are, or what sexual orientation you are. None of those things matter. You just have to be human.

I hear horror stories all of the time. I had one instance where a patient was going to a pharmacy which actually saw a lot of HIV patients in the community where the pharmacy was located. He went in one weekend and his ADAP had expired. The pharmacist came flying around from behind the counter, with a bible. The pharmacist threw the bible down on the counter, pointed at the patient, and told him he deserved what he got and there's nothing he could do for him.

You can imagine that the patient was devastated.

Another example: the patient goes in to pick up his prescription and is standing in line with the rest of the neighborhood for an hour and a half. He drops off the prescription and is milling around the store. The next thing you know they announce, "John Brown, your AIDS medication is ready." I heard that story just a few months ago.

You would think that doesn't happen anymore, but it's happening all of the time and people just aren't cognizant of it. Working in HIV, you are cognizant of HIV sensitivity and confidentiality every second of every day. Treat all patients with empathy and compassion. You have to be empathetic and compassionate. You can't just say, "You deserve what you got. Why didn't you call your refills in last month? What's wrong with you? Your ADAP has expired. Don't you know you have to re-enroll?" We don't know what our clients are going through. Unless you've walked in those shoes, you can never pass judgment on anybody.

Do not discriminate between ethnic groups or social classes. Every single patient should be treated equally. Whether the patient coming into your store is the CEO of the biggest corporation in the world or a homeless man who just walked in off the street, you should not treat those people differently. Also, do not treat patients according to their type of insurance coverage. Often people get so annoyed when somebody comes in with a Medicaid card and they say, "Oh, another one of those." It's very degrading to the patient.

We don't know why they're on Medicaid. With an HIV or AIDS diagnosis, the patient may be disabled and therefore have Medicaid. It is nobody's business and nobody should be passing judgment. Don't treat patients differently according to what insurance they have.

Patient confidentiality is paramount. Confidentiality is sacred. Treat all patients, while following the HIPAA guidelines, but especially with HIV. There have been so many lawsuits against pharmacies because of breach of confidentiality in HIV. Here are a few examples.

1. There was one case where the pharmacy technician went home and was talking around the dinner table. She made a comment and said, "John Brown came in today and picked up his AIDS medication." Her son and John Brown's son were best friends. The technician's son went to school the next day and told his best friend that his dad had AIDS. John Brown's son did not know about his dad's diagnosis. You can imagine the consequences that ensued, and a major lawsuit was brought against the pharmacy.

2. A woman came up to the pharmacy counter to pick up her prescriptions and the pharmacy clerk said, "Your husband's prescriptions are ready. Do you want to take them, too?" The woman said, "Sure, no problem." She picked up his HIV medicines. She didn't know he was HIV positive, and they were going through a very nasty divorce. You can imagine that the ramifications of the incident were catastrophic.

Stories like these happen all the time, so confidentiality is very important. You just don't get on the PA and say, "John Brown, your AZT is ready" or "Your AIDS meds are ready."

Consultations that the pharmacist provides should be done in a private consultation area. It should be a separate room away from the counter so that everybody else in the store and the community standing in line doesn't have to hear the conversation. Don't discuss or disclose an individual's HIV status. Derogatory or discriminatory comments should not be tolerated—ever. There should be zero tolerance for any AIDS phobia or homophobia in the pharmacy. It's just completely unacceptable. It's degrading to both co-workers and to patients.

Stigma still exists around HIV. We know that in different cultures there is a huge stigma. HIV pharmacies deliver to so many patients, and it's not as if you can just drive up to their house with a big sign on your van that says, "AIDS Specialty Pharmacy." We have to be very discrete. Many people live with multiple people in their home and don't want everybody to know that they're HIV positive. I have had many Latino patients kicked out of their house because people just don't understand. They really want to keep everything under wraps so that people don't know and so that they don't get evicted from their home. I had one client who lived in the back room of his sister's home, and when his family found out about his HIV diagnosis, he had to eat on paper plates. These stories happen all the time, even in this day and age.

When I educate and train new pharmacy clients who are just getting into HIV, they ask, "Can I get it if I touch the patient? Can I get it from using the bathroom, glasses or dishes?" You CANNOT get HIV from casual contact, touching an infected person, using the same dishes, glasses or bathroom. The pharmacy staff has to be educated and trained. The people working in the pharmacy have to know how to deal with HIV clients and be HIV sensitive.

As was mentioned in the previous chapter, the antiretroviral medications must be stocked and always be in stock. If the pharmacy does not have the drugs in stock, it leads to non-adherence and could lead to failure of the regimen. The pharmacy is then promoting the non-adherence of the patient. General pharmacies may be unfamiliar with HIV medications, and when a patient presents them with a prescription, they do not know what the prescription is for and definitely do not have the medications in stock. The prescriptions can often be misread and the prescription filled incorrectly. Here is an example: the physician wrote a prescription for AZT 100 mg. The patient went to a pharmacy that wasn't an HIV specialty pharmacy, and he got Azathioprine 100 milligrams. You can see that the results could be catastrophic.

Patients must feel comfortable and at ease at the pharmacy. All clients that go to these HIV specialty pharmacies are made to feel comfortable. When they call, people know their name and they feel welcome at the pharmacy, which is critical because of the stigma and discrimination many HIV patients face.

Be an advocate for the patient. You have to advocate for them. If something is not covered by their insurance, a patient would often go into the pharmacy and be told,

"This isn't covered on Medicaid." That's all the staff person would say. They don't offer to call the doctor, try to get it covered, do an authorization or just go that extra mile so that the client doesn't have to walk away and just not take that prescription. This was described in the previous chapter in the example about Joey. Being an advocate for the patient is also a critical piece. We all have to work together.

There are many laws that protect people with HIV. Those of you who have been around since the 80s know that people were getting fired from their jobs and evicted from their homes. We know the whole Ryan White story and what happened to him. You may have seen the movie, *Philadelphia*. Those were realities.

Having HIV is covered as part of the American Disabilities Act. It's also part of the Rehabilitation Act. In California there are great protections for people with HIV. Under the Rehabilitation Act, any facility that accepts federal funding for services cannot discriminate against people with HIV. There is also the California Fair Employment and Housing Act (FEHA) and the Unruh Act—which is the California civil rights law. There are also many local and city laws offering protections to people living with HIV in California—cities such as West Hollywood, Los Angeles, Long Beach, Pasadena, San Francisco, Santa Monica and Laguna Beach to name a few.

Laguna Beach is one of the only cities in the country that has an HIV advisory committee as part of the city council.

This was formed in 1987 to combat this massive epidemic that was going on in Laguna Beach. That committee is still going today and it provides incredible HIV education and HIV prevention services to the community of Laguna Beach. Educating youth and being allowed into schools to talk about HIV and HIV prevention (oftentimes a daunting task as the school authorities usually do not allow it) is critical in stopping the spread of HIV. The Laguna Beach HIV advisory committee goes to the high school and the middle school and the Boys' and Girls' Club to educate the kids and to talk about HIV.

That is the most impactful way to transmit that message to our youth—when they see one of their peers standing before them who has HIV and is telling their story and what they've had to go through.

I still hear horror stories of people in some cities where the landlords try to evict them because they find out they're HIV positive. These things go on all the time; our patients need to know that they have rights and that they are protected by stringent laws against these types of behaviors. This is another area where we can advocate for our patients and provide them resources where they can get help if they have been discriminated against.

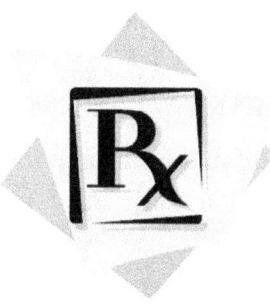

Chapter Four:
Marketing HIV Services

"Think big and don't listen to people who tell you it can't be done. Life's too short to think small."

— Tim Ferriss

How do you market your HIV Services and expand on your current practice or build your practice from scratch?

Marketing HIV services is different from marketing other clinical services, such as cancer or multiple sclerosis, because of all the stigma and discrimination people living with HIV have faced and continue to face today. Many Specialty Pharmacies have sales representatives that are out in the marketplace "selling" the pharmacy services to referral sources such as HIV clinics, physicians' offices, AIDS Service Organizations and also to HIV infected clients through support groups and other activities.

You cannot "sell" HIV services in the traditional sense with aggressive sales people who look at HIV patients with dollar signs in their eyes and have the "used car salesman" mentality, and each time they enter a clinic or physician's office, the staff run like hell. The HIV community is a tight, close-knit community, leery of newcomers. Physicians and providers are VERY protective of their patients and do their utmost in protecting them from predators and the "used car salesmen" that are clearly out there only to make money, don't particularly care all that much for their patients and only have one agenda—*make more money*, no matter what. The unethical and illegal activities that are conducted by many were discussed earlier in chapter one.

The "selling" and "salesman" mentality is off-putting to referral sources and HIV patients alike, and therefore, HIV services have to be marketed. You can only market your service when the "customer"—be it the referral source or patient—is comfortable with you, the pharmacist, as well as your team of people on the ground such as your community liaisons and reps who call on referral sources. They will only be comfortable once they know, like, and trust you and your team.

To be successful in marketing your HIV services, you must have "IT," and your team of marketing people that you hire must have "IT." "IT" is that thing you can't learn and you can't teach. "IT" is a mindset and a value that emanates from your core; "IT" is a sense of deep caring and compassion and commitment to your patients—the commitment to take care of them no matter what. HIV marketing is a "feel"; it is not something you can study in a textbook and then go out and do it.

Making a difference in your patient's lives is rewarding, and the side effect to providing excellent care with empathy and compassion is that your business grows and becomes more profitable. As pharmacists, we are looking for ways to counteract the shrinking margins, and through growing an HIV specialty with effective marketing you can overcome this issue.

Steps To Marketing Your HIV Services

1. Create a "Rockstar" TEAM

"Your TEAM is your greatest asset—teach them well." - Michelle J Sherman MichRx Consulting

The way to create a 'Rockstar" TEAM and make sure your HIV pharmacy is way ahead of your competition is to ensure that you have hired HIV sensitive, caring and compassionate individuals and make sure they GET TRAINED and get trained well.

See HIV Pharmacy Online Training at http://bit.ly/HIVRxTraining or scan the QR code.

2. BookUp your business

You're an expert right? You're an authority in your community and in your profession—right?

Well, the best way to market your business and showcase who you are, who your business is and what you do, is to become an author—write a book!

Everyone I talk to wants to write a book, but they don't because they think it's too hard.

Imagine if you had your book that you could give to doctors, insurance companies, AIDS Service Organizations and any other referral sources to get business; you would be LEAPS ahead of your competitors and business will come your way, guaranteed.

Want to get that book? Here's where to go: http://bit.ly/BookUpRx or scan QR code.

3. Create a marketing formula for your pharmacy:

The marketing formula will get you started from scratch, from the beginning, and must contain the following components:

- Your brand
- Your Unique Value proposition (UVP)
- Who your Target Market is
- Building an online identity through an online presence
- Social Media

An excellent guide that will assist you in putting these six steps together in a step-by-step manner is the book, *Care Your Way To Insane profits and Beat The Margin Game, A Pharmacists Guide To Modern Marketing* by Mitzie Sundberg, MBA.

4. Create a marketing plan:

Just as you have a business plan for your pharmacy, it is imperative that you have a comprehensive marketing plan in place to be able to effectively market your HIV Services. The marketing plan will be your blueprint for growing your HIV practice. Go to

http://bit.ly/CareMktgPlan or scan the QR code.

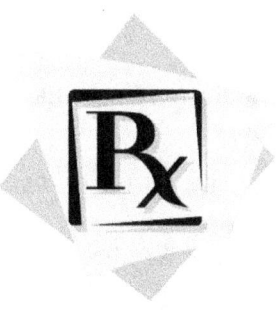

Chapter Five:
Insurance and Benefits

Dealing with insurance companies is the bane of every pharmacist's life. The amount of labor and manpower that is used each day on the phone with insurance companies or dealing with prior authorizations or insurance problems is enormous. The reimbursement rates insurance companies impose on pharmacies are shrinking and pharmacy gross margins are dropping. This is frustrating for many pharmacists and pharmacy owners. It is therefore important for pharmacists to implement programs and pick a specialty where they can implement programs, become healthcare providers, and improve on their bottom line.

In HIV Specialty Pharmacies it is imperative that the pharmacy staff are trained on how to deal with the insurance companies and how to co-ordinate the patient's benefits amongst multiple insurance carriers if they have more than one carrier.

Here are some examples:

- A patient has Medicare Part D and ADAP pays the copays
- A patient has private insurance and ADAP pays the copays
- A patient has Medicaid with a share of cost spend down and ADAP pays the share of cost

As discussed in the previous chapters, the pharmacy staff must advocate for the patient. If a medication is not covered by the insurance plan, call the insurance company. Come up with a solution for the patient; see what you need to do. Do the authorization for them. You can speak to the doctor if you need to, but as an HIV pharmacist, you should know what the patient is taking the drug for and do the authorization yourself. Send in the authorization to Medicaid, ADAP, Medicare Part D or whoever the insurance company is. Just take care of it. Deal with it for the patient.

AIDS Drug Assistance Program—ADAP

If patients qualify, the ADAP program may cover all or some of the cost of HIV/AIDS related medications that other insurance companies may not cover, or if the patient has no other insurance. ADAP is available in all 50 states and Commonwealths and the program is not the same in each state or Commonwealth. Each state is responsible for the following:

- Establishing ADAP eligibility

- Determining the type, amount, duration and scope of services
- Developing a list of covered prescriptions on its formulary
- Administering the program

ADAP is a payer of last resort, and funding for the program comes from both the Federal and State governments. The amount of funding that each state receives is dependent on the population of the state and the amount of people in that state that are infected with HIV/AIDS. States like New York and California, who have a large population infected with HIV, receive more ADAP funding than a state such as Utah that has a small population of HIV infection. States such as New York and California have robust ADAP programs with extensive formularies, whereas other states may have waiting lists for people to get onto the ADAP program. HIV patients have died while on the waiting list to get onto ADAP in some states, a situation that is unimaginable in this day and age.

List of states with ADAP waiting lists: http://bit.ly/UTBk8w,

or scan QR code.

Medicaid, The Affordable Care Act and American Healthcare Act

Medicaid is a program for certain people and families with low incomes and limited resources. It is a program that is funded jointly by the Federal and State governments and is managed by the states. To be eligible for Medicaid an individual must be a US citizen or legal permanent resident. Medicaid benefits may include low-income adults, their children and people with certain disabilities such as HIV/AIDS. Medicaid is the largest source of funding for medical and health related services for people with limited or no income in the United States.

The passing of the Affordable Care Act by Congress and the signing of the act into law by President Barack Obama on March 23, 2010, expanded affordable Medicaid coverage for millions of low-income Americans and made improvements to Medicaid and the Children's Health Insurance Program.

Provisions in the Affordable Care Act ensure healthcare coverage for all Americans, offer protections from health insurance companies and eliminate the pre-existing condition clause that has prevented health insurance companies from providing coverage to people.

While the Affordable Care Act is not perfect, it has had a number of successes and has saved countless lives. Here are some examples:

People Insured

- Pre-Affordable Care Act, 20% of Americans under 65 were uninsured.
- In 2015, the Americans under 65 uninsured dropped to 10%

Medicaid

- Americans using healthcare marketplaces who make less than $48,000 per year receive subsidies to help them buy insurance

- The amount of the subsidy depends on the income and cost of insurance in the person's area

- Subsidies are automatically applied to the person's monthly insurance bills rather than having to wait for a rebate

Insurance Mandate

- Americans are required by law to purchase health insurance or pay a tax penalty

Guaranteed Coverage

- All Americans can get health insurance even if they are sick. Insurance companies cannot deny coverage due to pre-existing conditions

Insurance and Benefits

- Insurance companies cannot charge sick consumers higher premiums

- Insurance companies can't impose annual or lifetime limits on coverage

- Insurance companies must offer a basic set of benefits, including mental health, prescription drug and maternity coverage

- Insurance companies may not charge older consumers more than three times more than younger consumers

This guaranteed coverage under the Affordable Care Act has been a game changer for people living with HIV. Prior to ACA, many people living with HIV could not afford insurance or were denied coverage due to a preexisting condition or did not qualify for Medicaid in their states.

These individuals relied on ADAP programs, which we discussed in the previous section and which are not so robust in all states. Some people living with HIV had no coverage whatsoever and many relied on manufacturer patient assistance programs or they just didn't go on meds, and got sicker and died.

Insurance Marketplaces

- Marketplaces such as Healthcare.gov and Covered California enable people who don't get healthcare benefits from work to compare plans

- All plans on marketplaces must offer a basic set of benefits, such as hospital care, prescription drugs and mental health services

Women's Health

- Insurance companies cannot charge women more than men for the same plan

- Insurance companies are required to provide a basic set of benefits which include maternity care, pediatric care and contraception

- Federal funding is provided to Planned Parenthood for family planning and other medical services used by Medicaid recipients. Abortion cannot be funded with federal funds

Taxes

- Insurance companies and medical device makers that benefit from new customers under the law pay more taxes

- Taxpayers with incomes above $250,000 annually are taxed more

So how does the GOP replacement healthcare bill, The American Healthcare Act, stack up? Well, lots can be said and debated, and regardless on which side of the aisle you sit, it's quite clear this GOP bill has no intention of providing adequate healthcare to Americans, and in my opinion is more a "deathcare bill" rather than a healthcare bill.

So as of June 28, 2017, what do we have put forth by Republicans in Congress GOP:

More Uninsured Americans

According to the Congressional Budget Office (CBO) both the House and Senate bills would result in major losses of insurance coverage that would affect mostly low and moderate income Americans.

This includes major reductions in federal aid for poor Americans who rely on Medicaid and for Americans who currently rely on federal subsidies to help them purchase private insurance through the marketplace exchanges.

The CBO estimated that in the House bill, 23 million fewer people will have health insurance over the next 10 years, and 22 million fewer people will have health insurance over the next 10 years in the Senate version.

How is this "Health Care"?

Medicaid

Senate Version:

- Will replace current Medicaid with a fixed per capita cap or block grant

- Each State would have a fixed amount of money every year. The amount would increase annually by a percentage linked to inflation rate, which is lower than in the House bill, resulting in deeper cuts

- Expansion of Medicaid benefits currently offered under the Affordable Care Act would be phased out beginning in 2020 and completely shut down by 2024

House Version:

- A fixed per capita cap or block grant would replace the current system

- Each State would have a fixed amount of money each year. The amount would increase annually by a percentage linked to inflation rate

- Additional federal funding that covered Medicaid expansion would be eliminated by 2020

My two cents: Both the House and Senate versions fail to actually take into consideration the health and welfare of those less fortunate than us, and instead of basing the program on improved health, welfare and care of Americans, the "bean counters" have literally made the lives of all Americans commodities on the ticker tape of Wall Street.

Now remember, this is just my opinion as a healthcare provider, a proud American and a human being.

Insurance Costs

Senate Version:

- Aid will still be linked to consumers income but it would be capped at 350% of federal poverty level instead of 400% under current law (ACA)

- A new formula for setting subsidies would tie them to the cost of less comprehensive healthcare plans, resulting in Americans getting substantially less assistance than under Affordable care Act

House Version:

- Americans would still get subsidies, but they will phase out at incomes of $75,000 per year

- The cost of insurance would be tied to a person's age, not income, so younger low-income Americans would get less help

- Subsidies would not vary with the cost of insurance, so Americans in high cost areas would not get as much help

My two cents: (This a DITTO of my comment above under Medicaid)

Both the House and Senate versions fail to actually take into consideration the health and welfare of those less fortunate than us and instead of basing the program on improved health, welfare and care of Americans, the "bean counters" have literally made the lives of all Americans commodities on the ticker tape of Wall Street.

Now remember this is just my opinion as a healthcare provider, a proud American and a human being.

Insurance Mandate

Senate Version:

- Eliminate the tax penalty

- Does not include any penalties for Americans who don't maintain coverage

Insurance and Benefits

House Version:

- Eliminate tax penalty

- Any American who goes without insurance for more than two months would face a six month waiting period to get coverage when they purchase a new plan

My two cents: I can understand the elimination of the tax penalty, but not the fact that under the House version that people who go without insurance for more than two months would face a six month waiting period to get coverage when buying a new plan—why? Again, this is a clause in a bill created by politicians who have absolutely no clue about health care and the plight of millions of their constituents.

Guaranteed Coverage

Senate Version:

- Would not explicitly eliminate guaranteed coverage BUT would allow States to seek waivers from several consumer protections

- States would be allowed to scale back conditions that they require insurers to cover, which could allow insurers to reimpose annual and lifetime limits on some coverage

- This Senate bill would not allow insurers to charge sick people more, unlike the House bill that does

- Insurance companies would be able to charge older Americans five times more than younger Americans

House Version:

- Would not explicitly eliminate guaranteed coverage, but would allow States to seek waivers from several consumer protections

- States would be allowed to scale back conditions that they require insurers to cover, which could allow insurers to reimpose annual and lifetime limits on some coverage

- States would also be able to allow insurance companies to charge sick people more, potentially making coverage unaffordable for some

- Insurance companies would be able to charge older Americans five times more than younger Americans

My two cents: WOW! Just imagine the impact this GOP insurance mandate would have on your patients—people living with HIV and older Americans. To me this really does sound like the death knell for many—higher costs because they are sicker or older or both.

Americans should not be penalized for having a preexisting condition; wouldn't you agree!

Insurance Marketplaces

- It is not clear how the marketplaces would work under either Senate or House bills because insurance companies may potentially offer health plans that do not offer the same set of benefits

My two cents: members of Congress have no idea how intricate and complicated the healthcare system is and have no idea how to "replace" ACA.

Women's Health

- Insurance companies would still be banned from charging women more

- States would be able to get waivers to allow insurance companies to drop some basic benefits, such as contraception and maternity care

- Medicaid would no longer have to offer maternity care and contraception benefits, which would greatly impact low-income women. Almost 80% of Planned Parenthood patients have incomes at or below 150% of federal poverty level

- Medicaid would be barred from providing funding for any health clinics that provide abortion services, including Planned Parenthood

My two cents: This is a complete war being waged against women—especially low-income women—by a group of men who have concocted a bill without input from women and with complete disregard to women's health.

Women's bodies are not vessels to be legislated against by men!

Taxes

- Insurance companies, medical device makers and wealthy Americans would receive a big tax cut as these taxes are eliminated

- Tax cuts total about $663 billion over the next decade

My two cents: All I will say is that these members of Congress who devised this bill are clearly bought and paid for.

So what is at stake for people living with HIV if ACA is repealed and replaced?

- Changes to Medicaid would have biggest impact for people living with HIV

- Changes to individual insurance markets will also have an impact on people living with HIV, especially with regard to pre-existing conditions, insurance rate setting, financial assistance, benefit provisions and administrative actions

- Ryan White program and ADAP programs will likely become more important for people living with HIV

See the report from Kaiser Family Foundation by going to this link http://bit.ly/ACARepealHIV, or scan this QR Code.

The Senate bill was due to go to a vote on Thursday, July 20, 2017, but the bill could not gather enough GOP support, was on life support for a few days and then died. Not enough votes to pass it.

My two cents: At the end of the day, regardless of one's party affiliation and partisan politics, it's quite clear that the health and welfare of Americans is important. This forms the foundation of who we are.

While the president continues to rant over repealing Affordable Care Act (for which there is no support), expecting the GOP to pass "something," the health and welfare of Americans should come first and foremost.

The Congressional Budget Office (CBO) has indicated that repealing the Affordable Care Act without a replacement plan will result in 32 million Americans being uninsured in 2026.

The Affordable Care Act is not perfect and can be made better in a partisan fashion. It has saved the lives of millions of Americans and the politicians in Congress who work for us should make improvements in a bi-partisan way, instead of coming up with new plans that are clearly ridiculous.

~~~~~

On July 25, 2017 the United States Senate voted to approve H R 1628 also known as The American Healthcare Act of 2017.

Vice President Mike Pence broke the 50-50 tie to pass the bill, setting in motion the wheels to derail the Affordable Care Act and strip millions of Americans of affordable health care and restrict women's health even more.

This was a procedural vote to set the stage for the Senate to start debating the healthcare bill from the House of Representatives. It will be interesting to see how this plays out and if the members of congress actually listen to their constituents. Keep an eye on what's to come.

Healthcare is a Right not a privilege

Watch the video here http://bit.ly/HCIsARight

or scan the QR code below

Medicare Part D

Medicare Part D has been around since January 2006 and is much more efficient now compared to the way it was when first implemented. For patients it is very difficult to maneuver through the Medicare website:

www.Medicare.gov, or sift through the mountain of paperwork on their own to determine what the best plan is for them. As healthcare providers and patient advocates, we can assist our patients in maneuvering through the Medicare enrollment process and guide them in the selection of appropriate plans for their needs, both in regards to prescription coverage and financial situation.

As pharmacists, we need to know what drugs are covered on the plan. If something's not covered on a patient's plan, we need to call the plan, try to get an authorization, see what we need to do and see if there's a substitute. Work with the patient; we are advocates for the patient and part of being a healthcare provider is solving the insurance problems. Never tell the patient, "It's not covered," and leave them hanging, because they won't know what to do and they may never do anything to acquire the help they need.

We must also be aware of coordination of benefits and be able to bill multiple insurances for our patients.

What will be the implications to Medicare in the American Healthcare Act if the legislation gets passed in some form? There are many unknowns, but Kaiser Family

Foundation issued a brief in July 2017 about the implications of AHCA to Medicare.

You can access the brief by going to this link http://bit.ly/MedicareAHCA, or scan the QR code below.

Private Insurance

Many of our patients with private insurance have high copays. For many patients, if they fit into the financial criteria, ADAP will pay the co-pays. If they do not qualify for ADAP, all of the drug companies for the HIV drugs have co-pay cards. Many of them cover co-pays up to $100 or $200 or even $400 per month for the clients. All HIV pharmacies should have co-pay cards on hand and offer them to the patients.

If a patient comes to the pharmacy for the first time, they are being checked out at the pharmacy counter, and they have copays, the staff in the pharmacy need to know about all these resources and try to make the cost for the patient as little as possible. Engage the patient: "Do you know you can maybe apply for ADAP if you make less than $50,000? (In California) Here's their phone number. Go make an appointment." "Hey, your co-pays are all adding up to $2,000. Use these co-pay cards." Even if you can decrease that amount by a few hundred dollars every month, every dollar helps the patient.

If medications aren't covered by the insurance plan, get them covered. If the HIV specialist physician is prescribing some-thing for a patient, they want that patient to have the drug that they prescribed. There's a medical reason for it. It should not be up to some attorney or accountant at an insurance plan to decide whether that patient needs that drug or not. We need to advocate on behalf of the patients in order to get the prescriptions that are prescribed for them and that will result in the best outcome for them.

> **"I go into more depth regarding insurance and benefits in a training video I recently made. I have included a transcript of the training video beginning on the following page." — Michelle Sherman**

Transcript of a video training session on insurance for the HIV patient by Michelle Sherman

This is Michelle Sherman, president of MichRx Pharmacist Consulting Services, bringing you HIV Training Module 6: Customer Service Part 2. In this training session, we're going to learn how to process HIV prescriptions and how to work with HIV patients and keep them happy.

"The best way to find yourself is to lose yourself in the service of others." This quote by Gandhi exemplifies what it is to be an HIV pharmacist and a staff member in an HIV pharmacy and how we can help our patients every single day and make a difference to our patients.

We come from a place of service to our patients every day. In that way, we're helping them. That makes us realize who we are as human beings.

The overview for today's training is that we're going to do a little bit of a review on customer service that we covered in Module 5. We'll also talk a little bit about pharmacist involvement and a brief medication review of items we discussed in Module 4.

We'll go through pharmacy workflow and navigating the insurance maze. Most of the time spent dealing with client issues is spent dealing with insurance issues. We'll talk about patient confidentiality and then do a summary of today's training.

On the customer service, this is just a little recap of what we did in the previous training session. Superior customer service is the cornerstone to helping patients. It is absolutely crucial that a high level of customer service is maintained at all times.

When a patient comes into the pharmacy, or even if they're on the telephone, always acknowledge them, even if you're busy. If you acknowledge somebody, they don't mind waiting.

They know that they don't appear to be invisible to everybody in the pharmacy. You've seen them, and they're happy with that. If there's a problem with reception and the patient is waiting, always inform them of what is going on.

Remember, if there is a delay in them receiving their prescription or they have to come back another day, if they know what is going on, they're apt to be fine with that. It's when you just leave them waiting in the front of the pharmacy for an extended period of time that will be aggravating and make them mad.

When people come into the pharmacy, they are sick. They don't feel well. They might have just been to the doctor and gotten a devastating diagnosis. They just feel sick, and they don't want to be kept waiting or left hanging, if you will. It's really important to go out there and let them know what's going on. That helps make them feel better.

Be polite and courteous at all times. Treat patients like you would like to be treated. Be kind, empathetic and sympathetic to their situation. Always be courteous. No matter how busy or aggravating your day has been, never let that show to the customer.

Follow through with customer requests such as easy-open caps. Are they going to pick it up? Is it going to be mailed? Does it need to be delivered? All those things need to be noted on the patient's file and complied with 100% of the time. Pharmacist involvement in the treatment of HIV patients is absolutely critical. We must treat patients with empathy and compassion.

When refilling the prescriptions, we need to try to fill all the drugs in the regimen so the patients get all the drugs at the same time. That's very important because some patients might not receive all their medicine at the same time. Therefore, they're not going to take the complete regimen. We need to follow up and make sure they get everything at the same time.

Getting their chronic meds and antiretrovirals at the same time every month cuts down on multiple trips to the pharmacy, multiple mailings or multiple times to deliver. Neither the pharmacy nor the patient is focused on getting drugs multiple times a month, so it's very nice for the patient and pharmacy to make sure everything is done at the same time every month.

It's very important to be sure to discontinue meds in the computer when the doctor changes the prescriptions. I've seen pharmacies not discontinuing meds many times. They just go ahead and refill the old regimen, plus the new regimen, and deliver it to the patient. There's no discussion or consultation that goes along with that and the patient just takes two regimens.

As you can imagine, that results in a lot of issues, such as exacerbation of side effects, toxicities and the like. It's really important that when a doctor discontinues a drug, that is noted in the pharmacy system and the medication is discontinued.

Prescriptions that are going to be mailed or delivered must be done in a timely manner, as patients can run out of the medicine and have their adherence interrupted. That is critical. As I mentioned before, there should be zero tolerance for the pharmacy-promoting non-adherence to a patient.

It's very difficult for our patients on a daily basis to be adherent with their meds. It's something they have to take every single day for the rest of their lives, so it's very important that we, as pharmacy professionals, take care of that aspect of it. We have the drugs in stock and make sure that they are filled for pickup, mailed or delivered on time so the patient never runs out of medications.

Patients that you have on auto-fill should be called every month to review the meds that are needed and to find out if there are any issues going on.

Another good thing to remember is to always double check addresses with patients. Sometimes they move and don't notify the pharmacy. When you're delivering or mailing, the prescriptions are going into an abyss because the patient is no longer at that location and you can't find them. It's very important to keep the demographics that you have on your patients up to date.

Always advocate on the patient's behalf. Whenever there are insurance issues or problems that go along with it, be the advocate for the patient. It's very difficult for them to maneuver through the system and try to get things done. If there's a problem related to their medication, the pharmacist and the pharmacy staff can then advocate on their behalf.

Most importantly, every time you're interacting with patients, remember that confidentiality is paramount. Even though we all comply and have the HIPAA laws in place, we really have to be cognizant of individual patient confidentiality when it comes to HIV patients, especially during phone calls and when mailing and delivering prescriptions.

How do you process HIV prescriptions?

Throughout the training, we've reviewed many things leading up to the actual filling of the prescriptions, how to address issues that go along with insurance problems and those types of things.

Just as a quick review from our previous training, this is the life cycle of the HIV. As a reminder, this is the six classes of antiretrovirals that we have. We have fusion and entry inhibitors, reverse transcriptase inhibitors, both non-nucleoside reverse transcriptase inhibitors and reverse transcriptase inhibitors, and integrase inhibitors and protease inhibitors.

The medications all act at these different sites in order to inhibit the replication of the HIV virus. That's what decreases viral load and maintains the integrity of the T cells in the immune system, allowing our patients to be healthy.

These are the approved antiretroviral agents in 2013. We have the nucs, the non-nucs, protease inhibitors, entry inhibitors and fusion inhibitors, and then integrase inhibitors that are currently approved.

What about pharmacy workflow? This is a critical piece in maintaining the efficiency of the pharmacy and ensuring that the operation works as a seamless engine to be able to deal with the HIV prescriptions and the volume of patients coming through the pharmacy.

Make sure the operations manual is available on HIV services. Within your operations manual, you need to create policies and procedures that directly relate to the provision of HIV services, where job descriptions are and how the patients are dealt with.

Make sure that the staff has read and is familiar with the operations manual. Beware of all job descriptions within the pharmacy, and remember that this is a team effort. Each and every person who works in the pharmacy, the pharmacist, technicians, clerks, drivers and anybody else, plays a critical piece and is a critical cog in the engine of seamless workflow.

You could do 100 prescriptions a day, and it could be like a nightmare. It could feel like you're doing 1,000 prescriptions because the workflow is not efficient. You could do 600 or 700 prescriptions a day with an efficient workflow, and by the end of the day you think, "Oh, my goodness. What have we done? We've hardly done anything today," and you have this massive volume.

Everything depends on the workflow, the training of the staff, and how efficient that engine is in the pharmacy. The workflow is the critical piece.

Make sure the pharmacy workflow is set up and efficient with an easy flow of dropping off prescriptions through the entire process, from the drop-off window or the receipt of a prescription over the telephone, from the fax machine or electronically, all the way down the line to completion of filling to dispersion for pickup, delivery or mail.

Make sure there is an easy flow of calling prescriptions through the whole process. You've got to make sure that everything flows and is a seamless cog that goes on inside the pharmacy and that the workflow is efficient.

Read the prescription

Carefully review the prescription and make sure the regimen is appropriate with regard to the combinations and dosages. Learn to determine conventional from unconventional regimens.

In Module 4, we actually looked at good regimens versus bad regimens. There might be HIV specialists in the area who, for whatever reason, have come up with a regimen for a patient because that's the particular regimen that's appropriate for that patient.

Remember that HIV regimens are highly customizable. They're customized to the specific needs of that patient. It's not cookie cutter where one size fits all patients.

Get to know the prescribers. Are they HIV specialists versus non-HIV physicians? HIV specialists deal with HIV patients on a massive scale and are experienced in treating the patients.

Non-HIV physicians might be inexperienced, and there's a greater likelihood of errors occurring or the prescribing of inappropriate regimens. You really have to be on top of this and monitor what's going on.

When you're standing there looking at that prescription, you have this tiny snapshot of the patient right in front of you. It's very difficult because you don't know everything that's going on with that patient. How did this doctor come up with this customized regimen for this patient?

You don't see that when you're looking right at the prescription forms, so you've got to ask patients questions about the other medications they're taking and try to get information from them as best as you can to determine if that is or is not an appropriate regiment. It is very important that you discern those things before you can move along the line and actually fill the prescription.

Insurance Coverage for HIV Patients

Now we'll deal with the big elephant in the room so to speak: insurance. It is the bane of everybody's life, I'm sure. We'll talk about Medicare Part D. We'll do Medicaid and ADAP and also talk a little bit about the Affordable Care Act.

This cartoon says, "Warning: May cause confusion, frustration, anxiety, hypertension, stomach upset and uncontrollable weeping," and the prescription is the drug plan. I'm sure each and every single one of you as well as all of your patients has gone through trying to swallow this pill of the drug plan and having all of these symptoms and side effects.

Dealing with the insurance companies is very challenging, so you need to set up systems, be aware of what all of the insurances are and what all their prior authorization procedures are, and be able to take care of your patients every single time.

The first thing is Medicare. This diagram over here shows the federal funding for HIV care in the United States by the different programs. This was from 2012 statistics. You can see that Medicare is the greatest proportion of this funding.

Thirty-nine percent of the federal funding HIV pie goes toward Medicare. That would be Medicare medical services and Medicare Part D prescription services. That is $5.8 billion or 39% of the federal funding budget for HIV.

The next thing is Medicaid. Only the federal portion of Medicaid, and not the state contributions toward Medicaid, was $5.3 billion and 36% of the total pie for federal funding on HIV.

Then we have Ryan White services which include things like ADAP and other Ryan White services at 16%, which is $2.4 billion. The next thing we have is HIV services through the VA at 6%, which is $.9 billion. Then there are these other federal funding services which are minimal.

The biggest pieces of the pie are Medicare, Medicaid and Ryan White. The total federal spending on HIV services in 2012 was $14.8 billion.

In this you can see the differences in the increases in federal spending for HIV between 2008 and 2013. In 2008 it was $23.4 billion and it has been increasing slightly every year since then, up to $28.4 billion in 2013. It increases every year because the number of people with HIV increases. We have 50,000 new infections in the

United States every year, and people are living longer as well.

HIV has become a chronic, manageable disease. Although it's very difficult and there are a lot of issues that go along with it, people are living longer and can have a nearly normal life expectancy, so you get an increase in medical care, pharmacy services and you have an increase in the federal spending for HIV services.

What are the different categories of spending for HIV services in the United States?

The biggest slice of the pie, which is more than half of the pie, is for care and treatment. That is $14.8 billion.

The next is the global outreach of funding. These are things like PEPFAR, the President's emergency plan for providing drugs to third-world countries and other global outreach for HIV services. That is 23% at $6.4 billion.

The next, at 10%, is for cash and housing assistance, which provides those services to clients living with HIV. That's $2.7 billion. Research is at 11% and $2.9 billion, and prevention is $0.9 billion and 3% of the pie. You can see out of all the spending that prevention services are the smallest piece of the pie.

When you think that HIV is 100% preventable, you would think that the prevention services and the funding for prevention would be a much greater slice of that pie. If we could prevent people from getting HIV in the first place, that's how we're going to decrease and end the epidemic, but it's only $0.9 billion and there are still 50,000 new infections of HIV in the United States each and every year.

Medicare

Here are some characteristics of the Medicare population. Many people with HIV are disabled and therefore qualify for Medicare, so you could get a 27-year old, a 32-year old and a 50-year old all coming into the pharmacy having a Medicare card because they're disabled due to the HIV and AIDS status. It's not just for seniors.

This is the breakdown of people on Medicare. Fifty percent of people have income below $22,500 and savings below $77,482. Forty percent have three or more chronic conditions.

Twenty-seven percent are in fair to poor health. Twenty-three percent have cognitive and mental impairment.

Twenty percent are dually eligible for Medicare and Medicaid, and many HIV clients fit into this 20% category.

Seventeen percent are under age 65 and are disabled, so many of our HIV patients fit into that category as well. Fifteen percent have 2+ ADL limitations, 13% are over age 85 and 5% are in long-term care facilities. You can see that HIV patients actually could fit into every single one of these categories.

This graph shows the increase in Medicare enrollment between 1966 and 2013. The dark blue bar shows people that traditionally are covered and eligible for Medicare, which are people age 65 and over. The light blue bar shows people that are not elderly disabled and they're under age 65, so that's the place where many of our HIV patients fall.

You can see that it seems like in 1966 and 1970 that Medicare was only for those 65 and over. From 1975 onward, people that were under 65 and were deemed disabled could then receive Medicare services. You can see here that it has increased significantly since then. It has gone from 2.2% to 3% and then in 2013 it is 9% of the people receiving Medicare who are under age 65.

This is a nice graphic showing Medicare beneficiaries as a percent of state populations in 2012. You can see in the light blue states that 10% to 14% of the population are Medicare beneficiaries and then it goes up. There is 15% to 16%, 17% to 18% and 19% to 21%.

Eight states fit into the category of the light blue 10% to 14%. Eighteen states fit into the 15% to 16%, and five states have the 19% to 21%. You can see in California that 13% of the population are Medicare beneficiaries. Florida obviously is really high. You have this higher population of seniors in those states.

You have other states like Michigan at 18%, Oregon at 17% and Arizona at 15%. This gives you a nice indication of the breakdown in the state populations in the Medicare beneficiaries.

Now we'll talk a little bit about the Medicare drug benefit and how it looks in 2013. For those of you who don't remember or who might be new to pharmacy, the Medicare Part D prescription drug plan only became implemented in January, 2006.

We're in our seventh year of Medicare Part D and there are slight changes that go on with it every year. For 2013 this is how it looks. When the patient is enrolled January 1, 2013, they have a Medicare Part D deductible of $325. During the initial coverage period which goes up to a limit of $2,970 in total drug costs, on average the plan pays 75% and the enrollee pays 25% of the co-pays.

Between the $2,970 and $6,733.75 is this blue area here, which is called the donut hole or the coverage gap. During this period, when a member gets prescriptions, the enrollee pays 47.5% of the cost on brand-name drugs and the plan pays 2.5%. Then there's a 50% manufacturer discount to Medicare on the other 50%. For generic drugs the enrollee pays 79% of the cost and the plan pays 21% of the cost.

All of the costs in this coverage gap that the patient is paying go toward what is called the true out-of-pocket cost. All of that adds up until the patient reaches a coverage limit of $6,733, which is called the catastrophic coverage limit. From then on the enrollee pays 5%, the plan pays 15% and Medicare pays 80%.

This is a basic overview of just a standard Medicare enrollee and the drug benefit. Many of our HIV patients are low-income individuals and they qualify for the low-income subsidy through Social Security. Many of these patients have lower co-pays during this part of the coverage as well as the catastrophic coverage because Medicare offsets those costs because of their low-income status.

With dual eligibles, for many of those they don't have any coverage or out-of-pocket costs during the donut hole or coverage gap. They, in essence, continue to pay their copays until they reach the catastrophic coverage limit. All of those are based on their financial abilities, so it could vary from client to client.

Again, this $6,730 also includes the true out-of-pocket costs for those patients.

Here's a little bit more on the low-income subsidies. Most Medicare beneficiaries with HIV will qualify for some type of low-income subsidy. The dual eligible, Medicare beneficiaries on SSI or Medicare savings program, which is called QMB, SLMB and QI, are automatically eligible.

Beneficiaries who aren't included in the group above but meet some income and asset criteria need to apply to Social Security or Medicaid to qualify for a subsidy. Subsidy accounts toward out-of-pocket costs and reaching catastrophic coverage level.

If you have clients that come into the pharmacy that have these high copays and they've signed up for Medicare Part D plan, in some instances they might not know about the low-income subsidy, if they've done it on their own. It's very easy to either assist them or direct them toward the Social Security website at www.SSA.gov. They can apply online.

One of the things I want to remind you of with your beneficiaries on Medicare is when open enrollment starts or they need to change a plan for a dual eligible, it's a great service to be able to sit down with the client, get on to the Medicare Part D website and try to help them figure out what will be the best Medicare Part D plan for them.

It's very difficult for patients to maneuver through this Medicare system and go online and try to figure out what is going to be the best plan for them.

As part of your advocacy and outreach, you can assist clients in selecting and picking the best Medicare Part D plan for them and their situation and all the medications and drugs they require for coverage.

We'll look at prescription drug coverage among Medicare beneficiaries in 2012. Forty three percent of the enrollees, which was 21.7 million, were Part D non-low-income subsidies. Twenty two percent were low-income subsidies. That was 11 million people. All the other Medicare enrollees, which was about 13.5 million, was 26%. Then 9% were employer-subsidized enrollees. That was 4.5 million.

We're getting ahead of ourselves here. I'm sorry.

Every state has their own Medicare Part D standalone prescription drug plans. Those are called PDPs. There are also Medicare Advantage plans which are more like HMO-type plans.

The PDPs, standalone prescription drug plans, only cover prescription drugs through those plans. All the other medical care and services the patient receives go through their regular Medicare.

States that are light blue have 23 to 29 plans, 30 to 31 plans. Thirteen states have 32 plans. Seven states have 33 to 38 plans.

You can see in most states, like Michigan, have far more prescription drug plans than a state like Alaska or Arizona. California has 32 plans. It just depends on the state as to the prescription drug plans that are offered.

This is the share of Medicare beneficiaries enrolled in Medicare Advantage plans. In the previous slide, these were the PDPs, the standalone plans. These are the Medicare Advantage plans, or MA or HMO-type plans.

Thirty six percent of Medicare beneficiaries in California are on these HMO Medicare Advantage plans. You can see that's pretty extensive in many states. You have Oregon, Nevada, Utah, Colorado and Arizona all here in the west that have very high enrollment in Medicare Advantage plans.

In states like Michigan, that's only 20% to 29%. Texas is 22%. New Mexico is 27%. Then there are just a few states, like Alaska, at less than 1% and Wyoming at only 4%. The New York, Pennsylvania and New Jersey area has a low incidence, as well as up here in the northeast.

That gives you an overview of Medicare, the breakdown of Medicare and Medicaid beneficiaries in the United States and how it involves our HIV clients.

What about Medicaid? The Medicaid programs are the state-run welfare programs, so to speak. A dual eligible has both state Medicaid and Medicare.

Medicaid

Each state has their own Medicaid program. In California, that's called Medi-Cal. That's what their identification card looks like.

Medicaid plays a critical role for selected populations. These are the types of people that have Medicaid coverage in states. We'll just go right down to here, the area that I've highlighted in red and yellow.

Fifty percent of people with HIV in regular care have Medicaid. Non-elderly people below 100% of the federal poverty level is 45%. Between 100% and 190% of the federal poverty level is 27%.

Medicaid covers a lot of families and children. All children is 35%, children below 100% of the federal poverty level is 70%, parents below 100% is 40% and pregnant women is 41%.

For the aged and disabled, 20% of Medicare beneficiaries are dual eligible, so they have Medicaid as well. Non-elderly adults with functional limits have 15%. Of nursing home residents, 63% have Medicaid. Many of them have Medicare also.

You can see that 50% of people in regular HIV care have Medicaid.

This is a slide on Medicaid enrollees and expenditures for 2009. You can see there were 62.7 million enrollees. The total Medicaid expenditures were $346.5 billion. You can see it's disproportionate. Most of the expenditures went to the lowest proportion of people.

Where the disabled population and people using it the most were 15%, they used most of the expenditures at 42%. Children, which make up almost 50% of the Medicaid enrollees, only used 20% of the expenditures. Adults used 14% with 26% of the population. Ten percent is for elderly who used 23%.

You see 35% of the Medicaid enrollees actually used 68% of the expenditures on Medicaid programs.

I've already mentioned that many Medicaid enrollees are dually eligible and have Medicare as well. Twenty percent of the Medicare population and 15% of the Medicaid population is dually eligible. You have 51 million Medicaid and 37 million Medicare enrollees. Nine million of those are dual eligibles. These are figures from 2008.

Dual eligible beneficiaries accounted for 38% of Medicaid spending in 2009. Just those nine million people out of the whole pie accounted for 38% of the spending, nearly heading toward half.

For the Medicaid enrollment, we saw 15% are dual eligibles, 10% aged and other disabled, 26% adults and 49% children.

Then for Medicaid spending, non-dual spending is 62%, long-term care is 25%, acute and others is 2%. Medicare acute care is 7% and 3% on premiums. That makes up the 38% of dual eligible spending. They make up 5% of the total population and enrollment but take up 38% of the spending.

Now that we understand a little bit about Medicare and Medicaid, we'll talk about the Affordable Care Act and patient protections under that act that's going to implemented in its entirety on January 1, 2014.

There will be coverage expansions to reduce the number of uninsured, health insurance reform to improve affordability of coverage and delivery system changes to contain the costs and improve quality.

The federal government will fund the vast majority of Medicaid expansion costs. Nine hundred and fifty two billion dollars, which is a 26% increase, is federal spending, and $76 billion will come from the state, which is an increase of 3%.

Those increases in federal and state funding to provide insurance for everybody will translate to 21.3 million enrollees and people having insurance by 2022.

There will be state savings, provided revenue and increased economic activity. This is all the impact of the Affordable Care Act and getting everybody insured.

The Affordable Care Act Medicaid expansion fills current gaps in coverage. We are going to have people that have no insurance prior to 2014 covered and be eligible for low-income health and insurance plans. It's getting coverage for everybody in our society.

Medicaid eligibility today is limited to specific low-income groups. You have the elderly, people with disabilities, children and pregnant women.

Then Medicaid eligibility in 2014 is going to extend to adults who are less than or equal to 138% of the federal poverty level. It's going to expand coverage for people who, prior to January 1, 2014, had no insurance coverage.

This is the current status of the Medicaid expansion as of May 30, 2013. These orange states are states that are not moving forward with Medicaid expansion, and that's 20 states. Eight states have an ongoing debate as to whether they're going to expand Medicaid. These dark blue states are 23 states, including DC, who are moving forward with Medicaid expansion.

States such as California, Nevada, Oregon, Washington, New Mexico, Colorado, New York and all these states in the Midwest are all going forward with Medicaid expansion.

States like Michigan, Arizona, Tennessee, Ohio, Indiana, Pennsylvania and Maine are debating whether that's going to happen. All these orange states have decided they're not moving forward with Medicare expansion at this time.

Other great features of the Affordable Care Act are eliminating the preexisting condition clause from insurances so everybody will be able to get insurance coverage without being excluded for a preexisting condition. That will be very helpful, especially for people with HIV who have up until now not been able to get health insurance. They will be able to afford that.

ADAP (AIDS Drug Assistance Program)

The last insurance plan we'll look at is ADAP, the Age Drug Assistance Program. Each state provides their own program to people living with HIV. It's a payer of last resort and takes care of people who don't have access to insurance or can't afford it and, depending on the state, fit into certain income criteria.

Currently, they provided medications to more than 226,000 people. These are numbers from 2010, and it has most certainly increased since then. In 2011, 58 jurisdictions received ADAP earmarked funding, including all 50 states, Washington DC, American Samoa, the Federated States of Micronesia, Guam, the Northern Mariana Islands, Puerto Rico, the Republic of Palau, and the US Virgin Islands.

ADAP has also received state funding and contributions from other sources, including other parts of Ryan White, but the support is highly variable and largely dependent on local decisions and resources.

ADAPs are not entitlement programs, and they are not payers of last resort. Each state operates its own ADAP, including determining eligibility criteria and other program elements, resulting in significant variation across the country.

Not all ADAP programs are created equal. Depending on where HIV patients reside, it could mean a difference as to whether they qualify for ADAP or they don't.

ADAP formularies also differ throughout the country. Formularies range from as low as 28 drugs offered in Idaho to 465 in New York. There are open formularies in three jurisdictions: Massachusetts, New Hampshire and New Jersey. You can see that there's a wide variety of different formularies and availability of drugs to patients, depending on where they live.

Insurance and Benefits

The majority of ADAPs, which is 30, covered every approved antiretroviral in each antiretroviral class as well as the one approved multiclass combination product.

Thirty-six ADAPs covered 16 or more of the 31 A1 drugs, which were highly recommended for the prevention and treatment of opportunist infection.

If you read the antiretroviral guidelines for adults and adolescents that you can get at www.AIDSInfo.nih.gov/guidelines.
It is a great document, and every pharmacy should have a copy of the guidelines.

This is a profile of ADAP clients as of June 2012. For race and ethnicity, 34% of the clients were white, 32% were black, 23% were Latino, 9% were other and 2% were unknown. Seventy-five percent of the male, 21% were female, 3% were unknown and less than 1% of the clients were transgendered.

Fifty-nine percent of ADAP recipients had an income under 138% of the federal poverty level. Nineteen percent were at 139% to 200%. Fifteen percent was 201% to 300%. Six percent had 300% to 400%. There were only 2% over 400% of the federal poverty level.

In additional eligibility criteria, the Ryan White program requires all ADAP clients to be HIV positive, low income and under- or uninsured, but no income level is specified under current law.

Each ADAP determines its own income eligibility as well as other eligibility criteria. All ADAPs also require documentation of HIV status.

This might sound very strange to you, but many people over the years have tried to get on ADAP programs and get access to HIV services such as social services, lower-cost housing, food stamps or services, mental health counseling and all the things provided to HIV patients through AIDS services organizations funded through Ryan White. That's why ADAP has required documentation of HIV status.

Every time a client enrolls, they need proof that they're HIV positive. In six other states, they use other additional clinical eligibility criteria. They actually want to see the CD4 counts and viral load ranges.

For example, in a state like California, they need documentation that the patient is HIV positive. Also, every time the patient reenrolls in ADAP, they need an updated viral load and T cell count on that patient.

All ADAPs have state residency requirements, and many require proof of residency. If you live in a state like New York and you want to enroll in the ADAP program, you have to show proof of residency. Many clients have to show proof such as an electric or gas bill.

Many clients don't have those bills or those types of things. They live with other people. In many cases, they would have to provide an affidavit stating that that particular client lives with them and is a resident of that state.

Finical eligibility ranges from 200% of the federal poverty level in 10 states to 500% of the federal poverty level in five states. Thirteen ADAPs also use asset limits to determine eligibility.

You can see geographically, depending on where you live, it will determine whether you qualify or you don't qualify for ADAP. This could have a great impact on patient care. That's why with the implementation of the Affordable Care Act, many people will have expanded access to insurance or even Medicaid coverage to be able to get into care and get medical services.

Many ADAPs have implemented cost-containment measures and waiting lists because of decreased funding and budgets in many states. ADAP funding comes from the federal government but also from the state governments.

ADAPs must balance client demand with available resources on an ongoing basis. As a result of recent economic conditions, instituting cost-containment measures, including waiting lists, has become increasingly necessary

This really impacts HIV clients in a very negative way. Over the course of 2011, 14 ADAPs had waiting lists, and waiting lists reached their highest point in September 2011 when 9,298 individuals in 11 states were eligible for ADAPs yet unable to access medications.

This is a dire situation for those patients. They're very sick. They're on a waiting list on ADAP. They have to wait for somebody to either die or get off ADAP before they can get on there. Many people have actually died while waiting on a waiting list to get access to drugs. When you look at the big picture, this is something that should not be happening in the United States in our day and age.

How does ADAP translate to Medicare Part D? There are 40 ADAPs that pay Part D copays, 34 ADAPs that pay deductibles, 25 ADAPs that pay premiums, and 40 ADAPs pay for meds in the donut hole.

As of January 2011, ADAP payments also went toward the true out-of-pocket costs. This is huge because many clients that have Medicare have copays, premiums and deductibles. For some of them who aren't dual eligible, they also have to pay for their medication in the donut hole.

You can imagine in 2013 when they have to pay about 50% of the cost, if they were on a drug like Stribild, for instance, that costs $3,000, where are they going to get the money to pay for the medication? It is very fortunate that there are 40 ADAPs that pay for drugs in the donut hole and who pay premiums, deductibles and Part D copays.

Usually the ADAPs will pay all these things, meds in the donut hole and copays, for drugs that are on their formulary. As we mentioned earlier, the formularies vary from state to state.

Hopefully this gives you an overview of how you deal with a patient when they come into the pharmacy as far as customer service goes, pharmacy workflow, and the reading, implementation and filling of the prescription, and of course dealing with all these different insurances and how they weave and connect with each other.

Many of our patients have coinsurance. They might have ADAP, Medicaid and Medicare. You have to maneuver through this whole thing.

We did not address in this training private insurance, but many patients that have private insurance, ADAP will pay the copays on those too, depending on the states.

In summary, in this training, hopefully you've gone through it and made notes in your worksheets for review at a later date. Remember that customer service is crucial. Workflow and operations is mandatory to the efficient running of the pharmacy engine to be able to take care of the patients.

Navigating through the insurance maze and having a good understanding about Medicare, Medicaid, ADAP, the Affordable Care Act, the ever fluid American Healthcare Act before Congress, and all coinsurance and coordination of benefits, is absolutely critical in being able to take care of your patients in an efficient, timely manner, and also being able to advocate on their behalf over and over again.

Then, of course, always remember the sacred rule about patient confidentiality. Remember patient sensitivity and coworker sensitivity. Advocate for the patients and solve their problems. Use common sense and good judgment at all times.

Most of all, have fun. This is a great profession that you're in, and you can make a difference in somebody's life every single day when you go to work and are helping your patients.

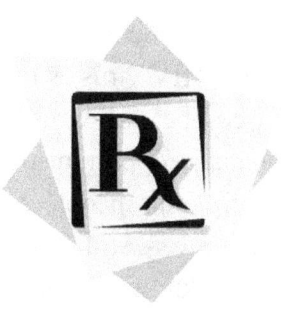

Chapter Six:
HIV Medication

History of Antiretroviral Medications

The HIV virus is one of the most formidable scientific challenges ever confronted. Back in 1981 very little was known about AIDS and how to stop or combat it. The CDC (Centers for Disease Control) first reported a "rare cancer" (Kaposi Sarcoma) among gay men. The first reports of KS came from Los Angeles, San Francisco and New York.

See report:
http://bit.ly/RiLbHq,
or scan the QR code.

In 1992 the diseases was defined as AIDS, and French scientists identified the HIV virus as the cause. There was no drug therapy to combat the virus, and all physicians could do was to manage opportunistic infections. AIDS clinics began to form and people were dying in the hundreds. In 1985 there were still no drugs to treat HIV or AIDS, very little was known about the mechanism of action of HIV, and there was very little support for patients who needed access to treatment. By this time there were 16,000 AIDS cases reported in United States and 20,000 globally.

In 1987, AZT (zidovudine, Retrovir®), the first AIDS drug, a Nucleoside Reverse Transcriptase Inhibitor (NRTI), was approved by the Food and Drug Administration (FDA). During this time there was the rise of AIDS activist groups, such as ACT UP (AIDS Coalition To Unleash Power), who held demonstrations and pushed for more rapid research and drug approvals to stem the tide of death. ACT UP demonstrated over drug price and access, and there were growing concerns over AZT toxicity and high doses that were given every four hours. Researchers began to test new drugs and look at twice daily dosing and expand treatment options.

Through the work of activist groups like ACT UP and the crisis of people dying, the FDA initiated programs for accelerated drug approval and early access. In 1991 a new NRTI, ddI (didanosine, Videx®), was approved, followed by ddC (zalcitabine, Hivid®) in 1992. In December 2006, ddC was discontinued due to side effects, toxicities, and the fact that there were more tolerable, less toxic alternatives available.

At the International AIDS Conference in Berlin in 1993, the Concorde trial showed no long-term benefit to early treatment with AZT monotherapy, and investigators realized that AZT monotherapy lead to rapid viral replication. Tests began on a new class of drugs, the protese inhibitors (PI), which would revolutionize antiretroviral therapy.

In 1995 the first protease inhibitor, saquinavir (Invirase®), and the first Non-Nucleoside Reverse Transcriptase Inhibitor, (NNRTI), Nevirapine (Viramune®), as well as NRTI 3TC (Lamivudine, Epivir®) were approved by the FDA. We now had three classes of drugs available to use, and the era of Highly Active Antiretroviral Therapy (HAART) began. HAART consists of three drugs selected from at least two drug classes, and HIV viral replication is inhibited at multiple stages of the HIV lifecycle. HAART transformed the lives of patients living with HIV and AIDS. I remember patients who were literally on their deathbeds, had all their affairs in order and were surrounded by loved ones, literally come back to life as a result of HAART. Patients now had a new problem to deal with—they had prepared for, and come to terms with dying, and now they were going to live. They now had to shift gears and start living again. This is known as the Lazarus Syndrome. By 1996 U.S. AIDS deaths fell for the first time, and many patients regained good health and were able to return to work.

As people began to "live," their *quantity of life* was extended, but the *quality of life* was impacted. There was a high pill burden, with dietary restrictions. It was the norm for patients to be on twenty, thirty or more medications each day. Side effects started to become a particular concern, especially lipo-dystrophy. Other side effects of concern were dry skin, nail abnormalities, kidney stones, allergic reactions and also metabolic abnormalities such as increased lipids and diabetes.

In 1997 antiretroviral switching emerged as a trend, and physicians began switching patients from one PI to another, based on convenience, efficacy and tolerability. Switches were from saquinavir (Invirase®) to indinavir (Crixivan®) and also to nelfinavir (Viracept®) and ritonavir (Norvir®). The second NNRTI, delavridine (Rescriptor®), was also approved. During this time it became apparent that there were adherence challenges for patients, and studies showed that a high level of adherence (95% or greater) was important to reduce drug resistance and treatment failure. The regimens our patients were taking were complex and gave them major adherence challenges. Drug manufacturers were working to create drugs that could be dosed less frequently, looking at once-daily regimes instead of twice-daily regimens and also the possibility of co-formulated medications containing more than one medication to help with pill burden and improve adherence. Combivir® was the first co-formulated product containing AZT and lamivudine.

In 1998 the third NNRTI and first once-daily antiretroviral formulation was approved, efavirenz (Sustiva®), as well as a new NRTI, abacavir (Ziagen®). 1999 saw the approval of a new protease inhibitor, amprenavir (Agenerase®), and in 2000, three products were approved: a new protease inhibitor that was the first combination protease inhibitor containing lopinavir, low dose ritonavir (Kaletra©), as well as a once daily reformulation of ddI (Videx EC®). The second co-formulation product was also approved, zidovudine/lamivudine/abacavir (Trizivir®). In 2001 the NRTI tenofovir (Viread®), a once daily formulation was approved, and in 2002 three reformulations of drugs were approved, which made dosing simpler by decreasing pill burden and helped to improve patient adherence. The reformulations were efavirenz-600mg (Sustiva®), Lamivudine 300mg (Epivir®) dosed once daily, and stavidine once daily (Zerit XR®). Zerit XR® never actually made it to the pharmacy and general circulation for patient use.

In 2003 four new medications were approved; enfurvitide (Fuzeon®), which was the first entry inhibitor to treat HIV, administered by injection twice daily. Two new protease inhibitors were approved: fosamprenavir (Lexiva®), given once or twice a day and atazanavir (Reyataz®), given once a day. A new NRTI, emtricitabine (Emtriva®) was also approved. Nelfinavir (Viracept®) was reformulated to decrease pill burden to a 625mg dosage form. The switching trend was fueled by increased options, and physicians were looking at protease inhibitor sparing regimens to improve convenience and reduce lipodystrophy. Once daily NRTI's were increasingly seen as alternatives to twice daily dosing.

In 2004 two co-formulated products were approved, lamivudine/abacavir (Epzicom®) and tenofovir/emtricitabine (Truvada®). In 2005 a new protease inhibitor, tipranavir (aptivus®), was approved and saquinavir (Invirase®) was reformulated to 500 mg tablet formulation.

In 2006 two drug manufacturers collaborated for the first time ever—Bristol Myers Squibb and Gilead Sciences—to bring to market the first once-a-day single tablet regimen, Atripla®, which was a co-formulation of tenofovir/emtricitabine/ efavirenz. The approval of Atripla® revolutionized antiretroviral therapy and gave providers and patients alike the hope of simpler more tolerable antiretroviral regimens that would help with patient adherence. A new protease inhibitor, darunavir (Prezista®) was also approved.

2007 was a great year for the approval of new therapies. A new NNRT etravirine (Intelence®) was approved. Intelence® had a different resistance profile to the three other approved NNRTI's and gave hope for patients who had failed therapy and had blown the NNRTI class due to resistance. The next generation entry inhibitor, maraviroc (Selzentry®), was approved as well as a drug, raltegravir (Maraviroc®) in a new fourth class of antiretroviral agents—the integrase inhibitors. The approval of these agents was groundbreaking, especially for patients who were on salvage therapies, who had multidrug resistance and were just waiting for new therapies to come along that would work for them and save their lives. Many patients with multidrug resistance who had never reached an undetectable viral load, and were on many antiretroviral agents, now had an arsenal of agents that were all approved within the same year, and they could start regimens with three new drugs at the same time. For many patients the results were remarkable and they were able to, for the first time, reach an undetectable viral load.

In 2011 a new NNRTI, rilpivirine (Edurant®), was approved as well as the second single tablet regimen Complera® (tenofovir/emtricitabine/rilpivirine). A once-daily single tablet of nevirapine (Viramune XR®) was also approved.

In 2012 the FDA approved the "Quad," Stribild® (tenofovir/emtricitabine/elvitegravir/cobicistat), which is a single tablet regimen containing four agents. Elvitegravir is a new generation integrase inhibitor, and cobicistat is a new boosting agent. Unlike ritonavir, cobicistat works as a boosting agent (it boosts the drug levels of elvitegravir), but it does not have the drug-drug interaction issues that go along with ritonavir.

In 2012 the FDA also approved Truvada® (emtricitabine/tenofovir alafenamide) for use as pre-exposure prophylasis (PrEP) in high-risk HIV negative people.

Pharmacists can play a very important role in HIV prevention and PrEP is a perfect situation for us to be involved in HIV testing, provision of Truvada® for PrEP and counseling on Truvada® as well followup HIV testing.

At the end of this section on meds I will give you QR codes and links to the current PrEP guidelines and the PrEP Clinical Providers Supplement.

In August 2013 the FDA approved dolutegravir (Tivicay®), and in August 2014 the single tablet regimen Triumeq ® (abacavir/lamivudine/dolutegravir) was approved.

In September 2014 the FDA approved cobicistat (Tybost®) and elvitegravir (Vitekta®). Cobicistat is a pharmacokinetic enhancer used to boost drug levels of other antiretrovirals, just as we have been using ritonavir (Norvir®) as a boosting agent for many years.

In October 2016, Gilead Sciences, the manufacturer of Vitekta®, made a business decision to permanently discontinue manufacturing the drug. The discontinuation was not related to safety or efficacy of the drug, but it was a product that was not widely used.

Since cobicastat was an efficacious boosting agent, the FDA approved two new medication combinations in January 2015. The first was Prezcobix® (darunavir/cobicistat) and the second was Evotaz® (atazanavir/cobicistat). Both of these new formulations eliminated the need for ritonavir (Norvir®) to be used as a boosting agent for both atazanavir (Reyataz®) and darunavir (Prezista®) (that's the 800mg once daily dose of darunavir).

In November 2015 FDA approved Gilead Sciences' single tablet regimen Genvoya®. Gilead had been working on a new formulation of tenofovir. The current version of tenofovir prior to November 2015 was tenofovir disoproxil 300mg.

Tenofovir is a drug that is predominantly excreted by the kidney and over time some people living with HIV who were on tenofovir containing regimens had decreases in their kidney function and progression of kidney disease, as well as increased bone loss and risk of osteopenia and osteoporosis.

The new formulation of tenofovir approved for use in the new formulation Genvoya® (TAF/emtricitabine/elvitegravir/cobicistat) was tenofovir alafenamide. Neither TDF (tenofovir disoproxil) or TAF (tenofovir alafenamide) can get into peripheral blood moninuclear cells (PBMC's), which also include lymphocytes. Only the tenofovir itself can get into these cells.

Both TAF & TDF are prodrugs and are converted into tenofovir in the plasma. 10 percent of tenofovir from TDF gets ito PBMC's and 90 percent is excreted via kidneys. 90 percent of tenofovir from TAF gets into PBMC's and 10 percent is excreted via kidneys.

As a result, lower doses of TAF (25mg) are used versus TDF 300mg. Studies have also shown TAF does not have the same bone loss as TDF and also has better renal outcomes.

In March 2016 FDA approved Odefsey® (TAF/emtricitabine/rilpivarine) and in April 2016 FDA approved Descovy® (TAF/emtricitabine).

Currently, seven antiretroviral drugs have been approved in generic formulation in United States: AZT, lamivudine, didanosine, stavudine, nevirapine and abacavir and the first generic lopinavir/ritonavir. As of the publication of this second addition of the book, only the liquid formulation of lopinavir/ritonavir is available and not the tablets....yet.

Three coformulated products are now available in generic: abacavir/lamivudine/AZT, abacavir/lamivudine and azt/lamivudine.

So now what about new HIV treatments in the pipeline? Here we go:

- Doravarine is an NNRTI that is potent at low doses and has fewer adverse effects compared to efavirenz

- Cabotegravir is an exciting new integrase inhibitor similar to dolutegravir. Cabotegravir is a nano-technology formulation and has a half-life of 21 to 50 days. This drug is being studied as an injectable with intra muscular administration. Dosing is being looked at monthly or quarterly, and maintenance therapy in combination with rilpivirine. Cabotegravir is also being looked at as an agent for PrEP (pre-exposure prophylaxis)

- GS-9883, also known as bictegravir, is an integrase inhibitor currently in phase III clinical trials as part of a fixed dose combination of bictegravir/emtricitabine/ tenofovir alafenamide)

- GS-CA1 is a new novel class of drugs called a capsid inhibitor

- BMS-663068 (Fostemsavir) is a CD4+ attachment inhibitor. It is a new class of drug especially for patients with multi-drug resistant virus. It is a pro-drug of BMS-626528 that inhibits CD4+ binding by itself to thegp120 protien on HIV. Studies are ongoing.

- BMS-955176 is a maturation inhibitor and is a new class of drug that would stop maturation of new copies of HIV virus. Another maturation inhibitor, beverimat, was studied, but 50% of patients had polymorphisms. BMS-955176 is a second-generation maturation inhibitor that has shown a better resistance profile. Studies are ongoing.

- Dolutegravir/rilpivirine combination has been submitted to FDA for approval.

- The first protease inhibitor fixed dose single tablet regimen combination darunavir/cobicistat/emtricitabine/tenofovir alafenamide has been submitted to FDA for approval

Through this history of antiretroviral therapy, you can see how far we have come in such a short period of time—from a time when we were helpless and had nothing to combat the HIV virus, to a robust arsenal with simpler, more tolerable, regimens and with several agents with new target sites in the pipeline.

If you have not done so already, I highly recommend that you download the Adult and Adolescent Guidelines, which provide extensive guidance on when to start, what to start, drug-drug interactions and adherence.

The HIV guidelines are continually updated. Get them at this link: http://aidsinfo.nih.gov/guidelines/, or scan the QR code.

Remember, a few pages back I promised the guidelines and provider supplement on PrEP…well here it is.

PrEP Guidelines go to this link http://bit.ly/PrEPGuide or scan the QR code below.

For the PrEP Clinical Providers' Supplement go to this link http://bit.ly/PrEPSupplement or scan the QR code below.

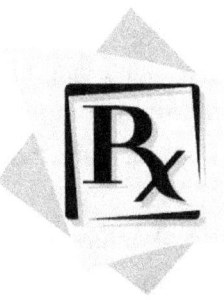

Chapter Seven:
Putting It All Together

"A person with ubuntu is open and available to others, affirming of others, does not feel threatened that others are able and good, for he or she has a proper self-assurance that comes from knowing that he or she belongs in a greater whole and is diminished when others are humiliated or diminished, when others are tortured or oppressed."

– Desmond Tutu

Only a few years ago, little hope existed for the effective treatment of HIV disease. Once diagnosed, individuals had few, if any, therapeutic options. There has been tremendous advancement in drug therapies for HIV disease in the past few years, and individuals who were dying now have the chance to lead healthier, productive lives.

While providing tremendous benefits, new HIV/AIDS drug therapies can also make significant demands on individuals due to their often-complicated regimens and possible side effects. Not only are individuals frequently at higher risk for adverse drug reactions, drug-drug interactions and drug-food interactions, but inconsistent adherence with drug therapies can jeopardize their HIV treatment altogether. Non-adherence to drug therapy is directly correlated with the development of antiretroviral resistance, leading to treatment failure as well as the emergence of multi-drug resistant virus. The development of drug resistant strains of HIV not only reduces the individual's chance for subsequent therapeutic success, but also poses a potential public health risk if an individual spreads resistant viruses to others. The care of HIV disease is a chronic maintenance disease where community-based resources are critical for success.

Given these issues, pharmacist involvement in the care of HIV infected individuals is critical, especially in the areas of drug therapy counseling, drug interaction monitoring, and adherence. HIV treatment failure is related to problems with patient adherence to drug therapy and with drug potency. Many patients have been HIV infected for many years, and the challenges of "lifetime adherence" become increasingly difficult as patients face pill fatigue and long-term toxicities from the medications.

As has been shown in the chapters of this book, the pharmacist has become a key member of a patient's healthcare team, and can be, and should be, instrumental in the management of drug therapies, resulting in improved patient outcomes and quality of life and lower healthcare costs. We became pharmacists to help patients; we are healthcare providers, and there is nothing more rewarding than being able to make a significant impact in the lives of our patients—it is a matter of *Saving Lives.*

I go into each day and to the care of my patients with the spirit of *Ubuntu.* Ubuntu is a quality that originated from the Xhosa and Zulu tribes in South Africa; it is a quality that includes the human virtues of compassion and humanity. What happens to you, happens to me, and happens to all of us. Adopt the spirit of Ubuntu in your pharmacy practice and it will forever change your life.

*"Do your little bit of good where you are;
it's those little bits of good put together that overwhelm
the world."*

— Desmond Tutu

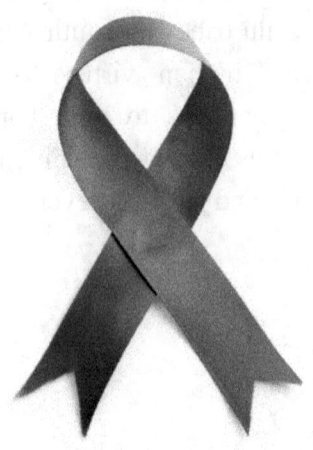

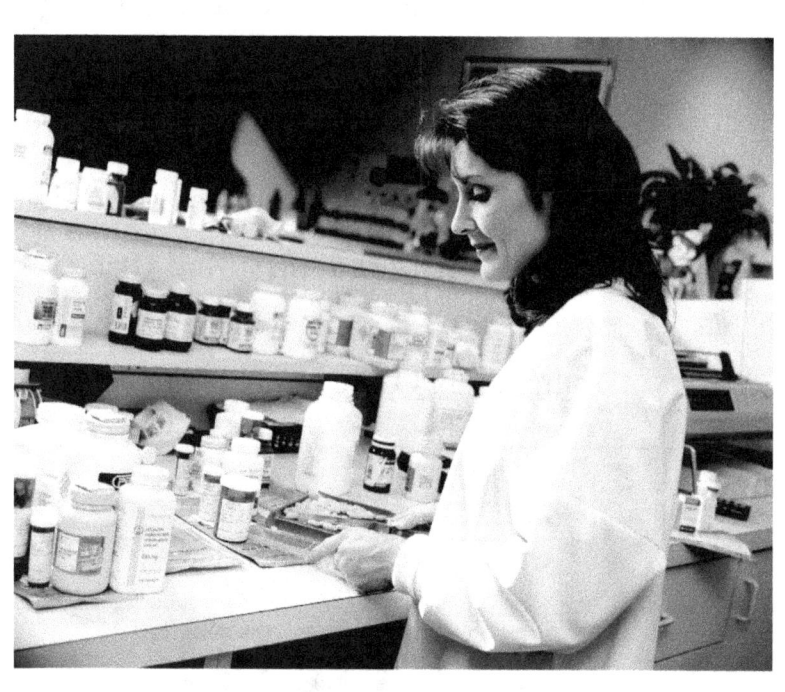

FREE Stuff From MichRx Consulting

Sick of Mandatory Mail Order Mandates?

Go to the Link below to Download our Article

"Overcoming Mandatory Mail Order"

http://bit.ly/OvercomingMailOrder

Or Scan the QR Code Below

Crush Mail Order Mandates With Tech

Go to the Link below to Download our

E-Book

**"Using Technology To Crush Mandatory
Mail Order Mandates"**

http://bit.ly/CrushMailOrder

Or Scan the QR Code below

About the Author

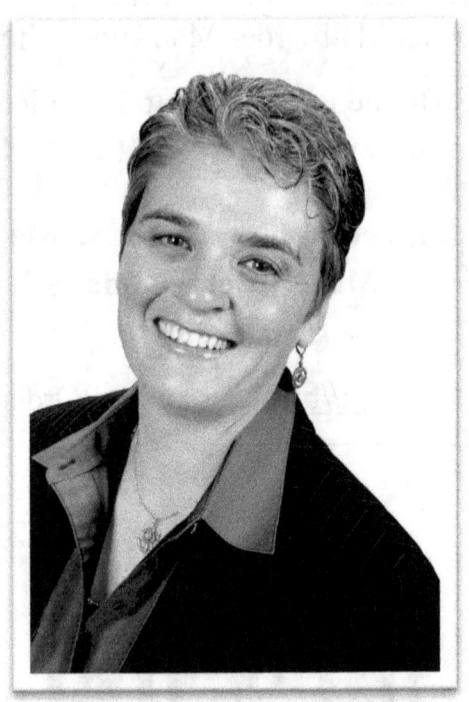

66 **A**s far back as I can remember, growing up in South Africa, one thing was always obvious to me. It was something that emanated from my core, from my soul, if you will. It was the "knowing" that all human beings are created equal, that we are all the same. I had this overwhelming drive to help people."

Michelle is is an author, speaker, consultant and advisor, and as a pharmacy entrepreneur and innovator, Michelle has developed a leading edge Medication Therapy Management program: Ubuntu Pharmacist Care Program, saving lives and managing drug therapies and outcomes for people living with HIV.

Michelle is committed to advancing the recognition of pharmacists as key healthcare providers on a patient's care team. To achieve this she has a non-profit organization, The Center For Advanced Pharmacist Care, to further advance and recognize medication therapy management within the healthcare system.

For FREE Access To the eBook, "Using Technology To Crush mandatory Mail Order Mandates"

Visit: http://bit.ly/CrushMailOrder

www.ingramcontent.com/pod-product-compliance
Lightning Source LLC
Chambersburg PA
CBHW070702290526
45790CB00001B/414